Gastritis - New Approaches and Treatments

Edited by Bruna Maria Roesler

Published in London, United Kingdom

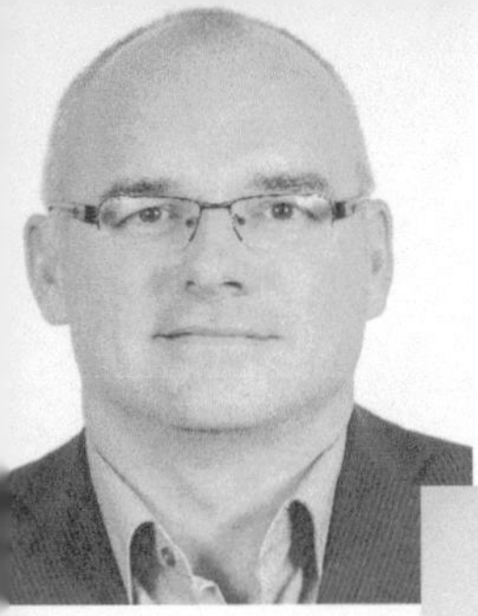
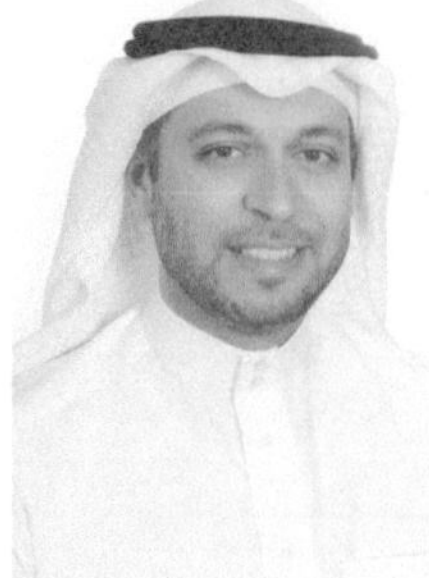
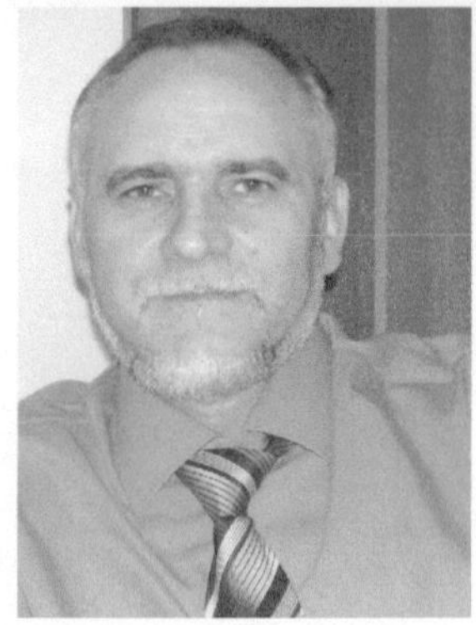
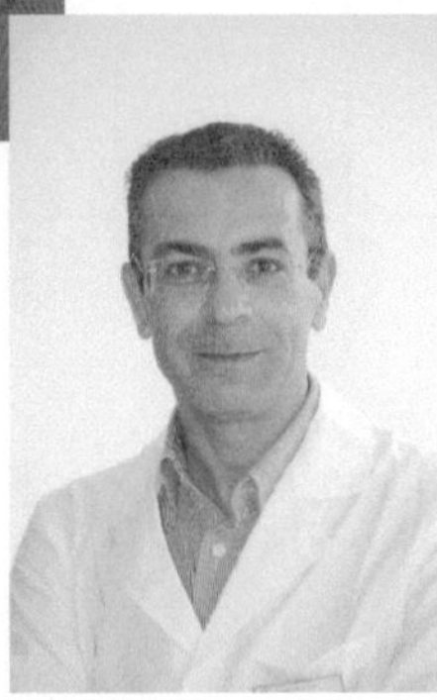
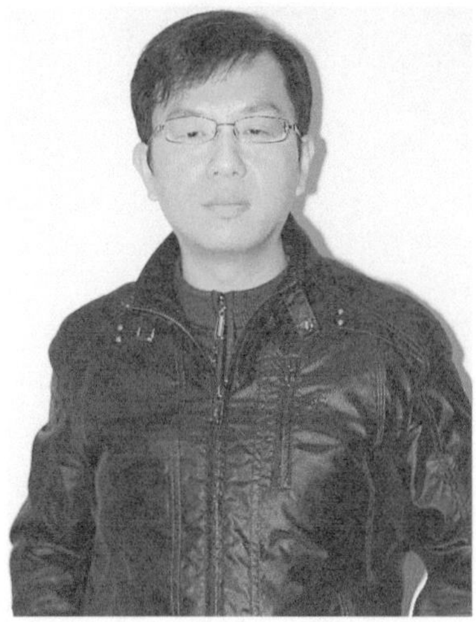
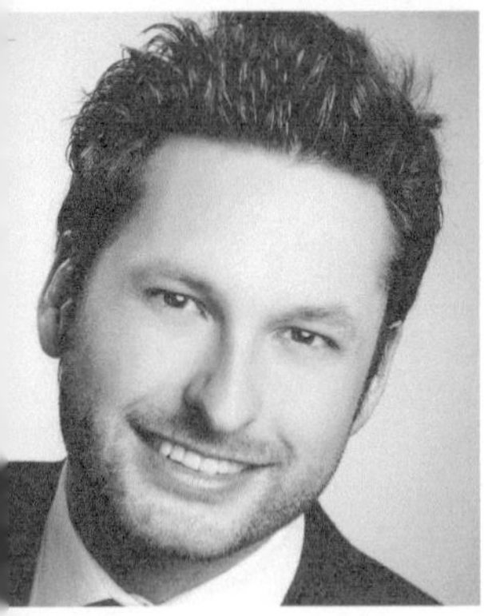
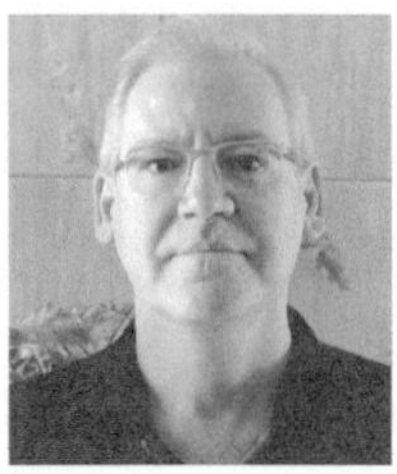

IntechOpen

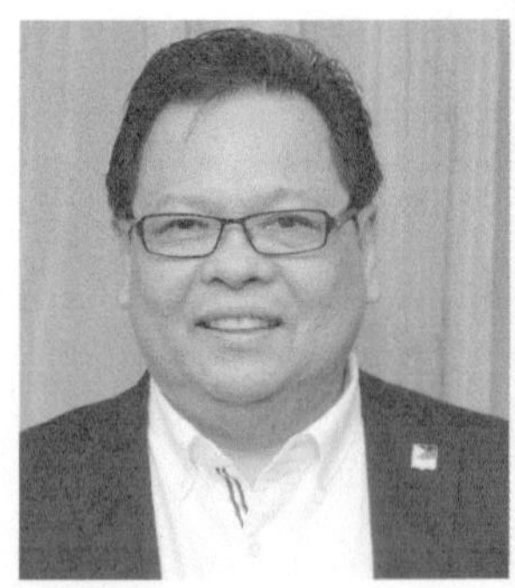
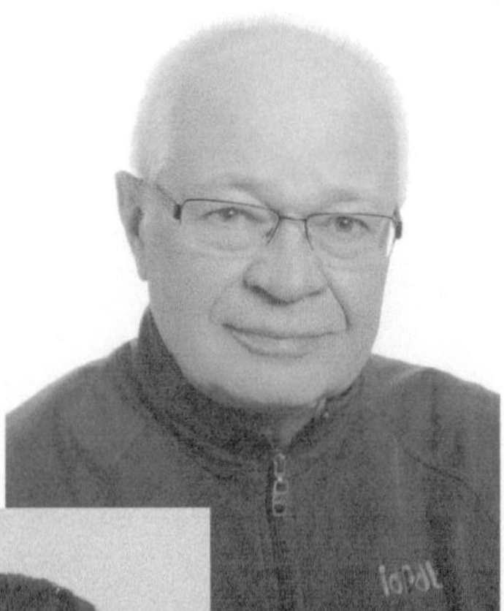
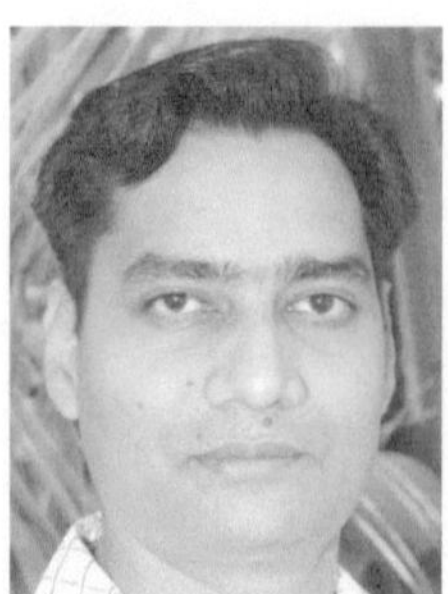
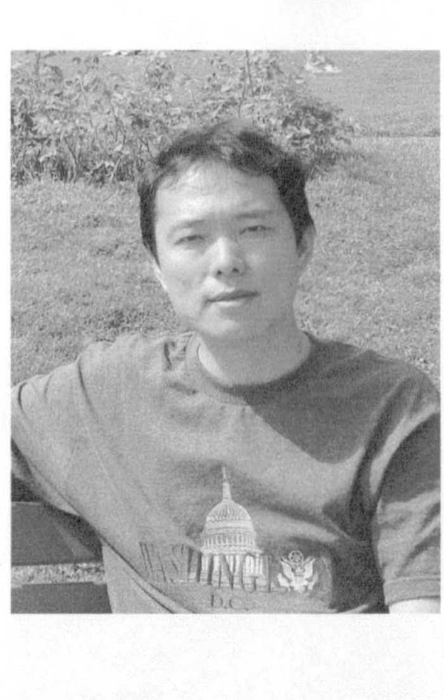
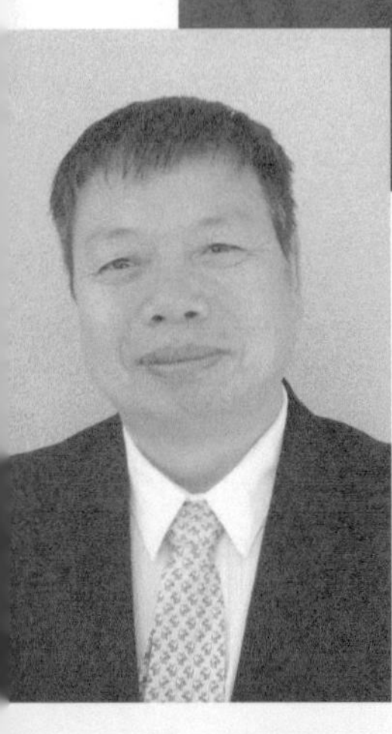
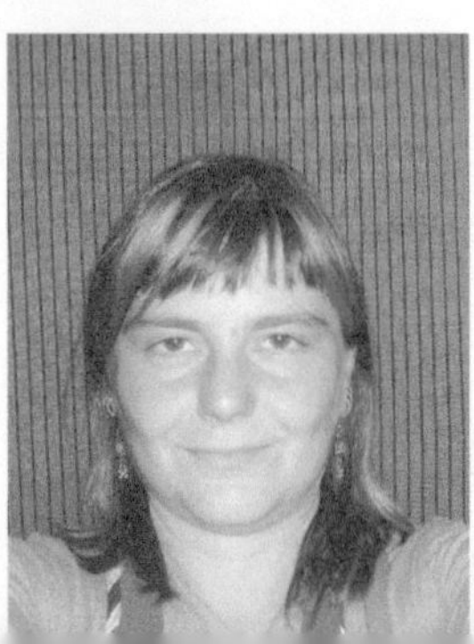

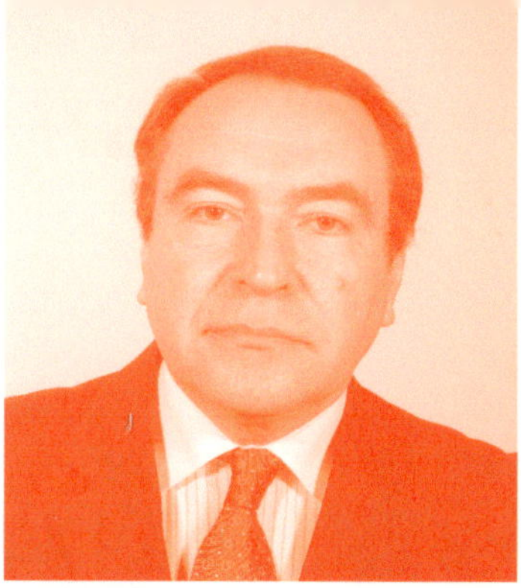
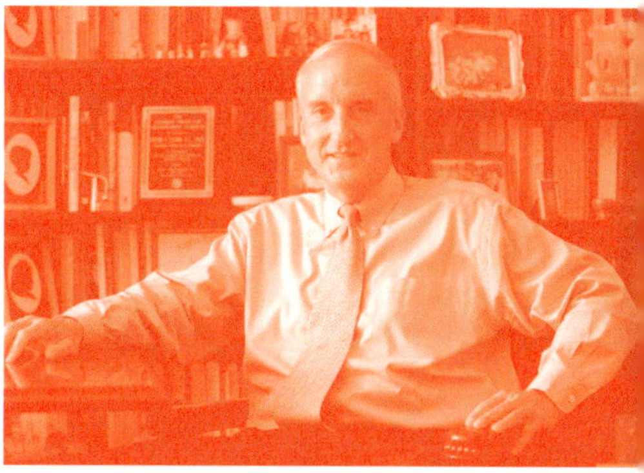
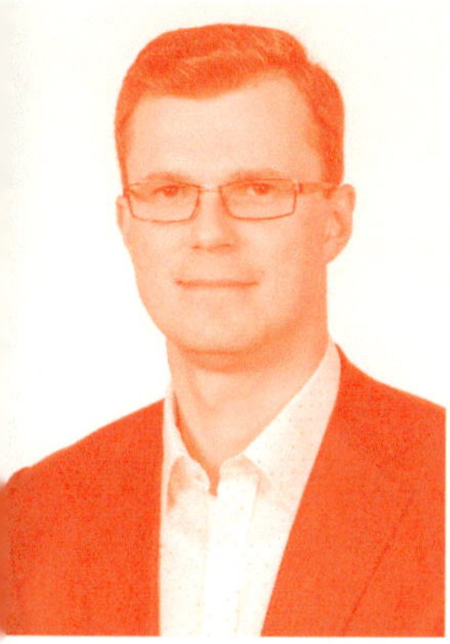
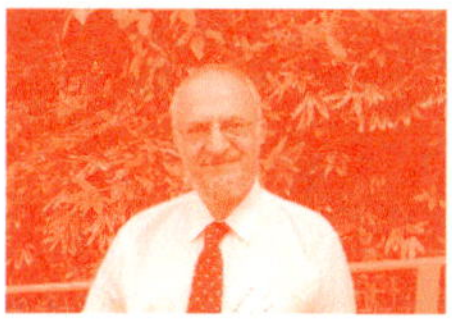
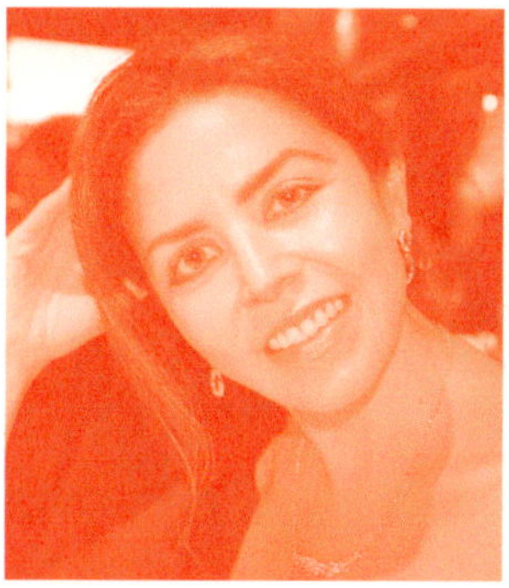

Supporting open minds since 2005

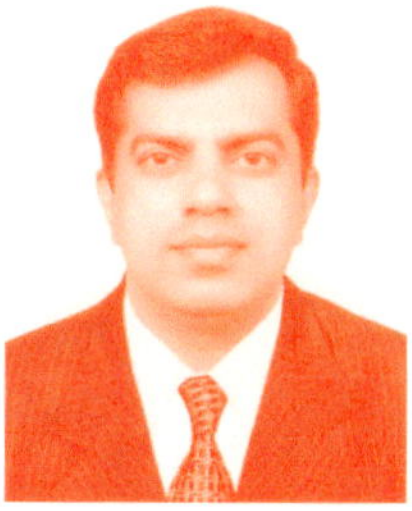
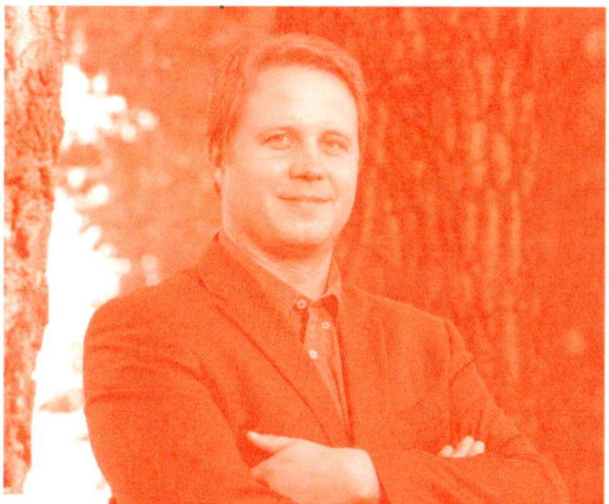
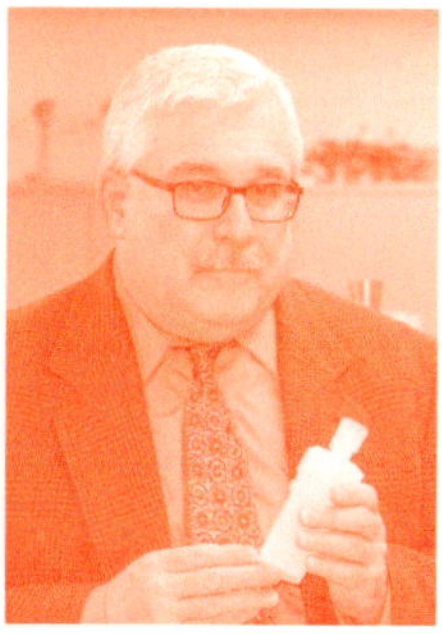
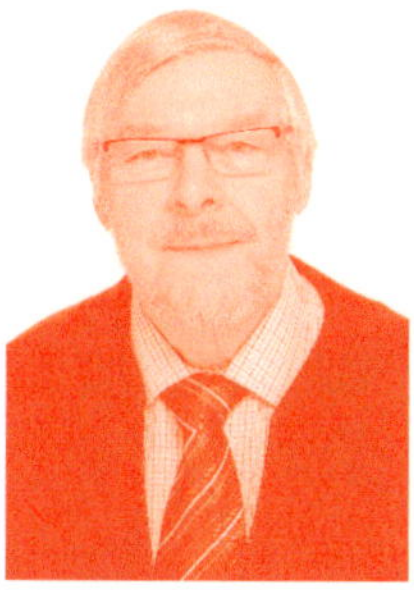
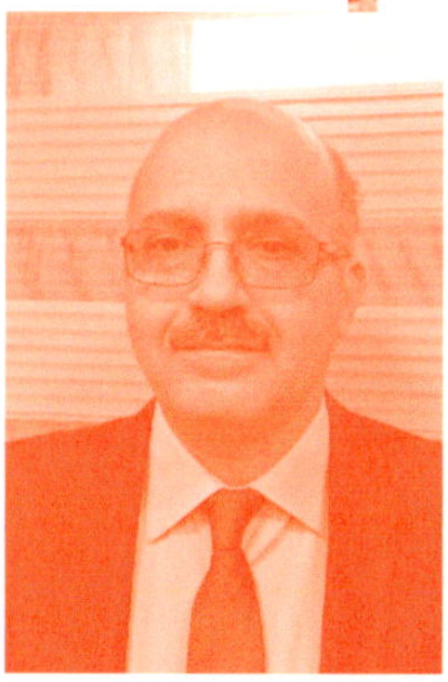
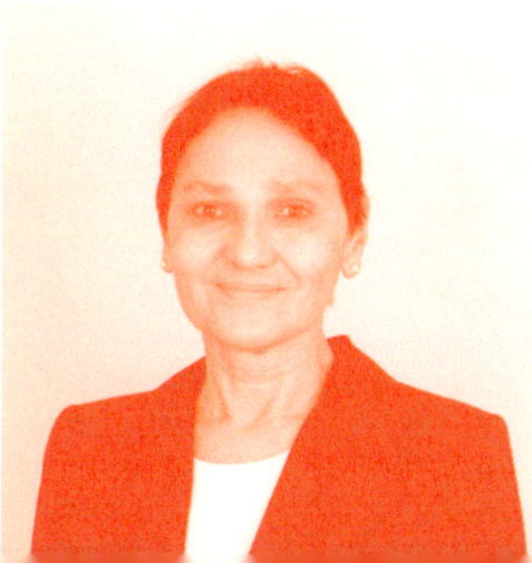
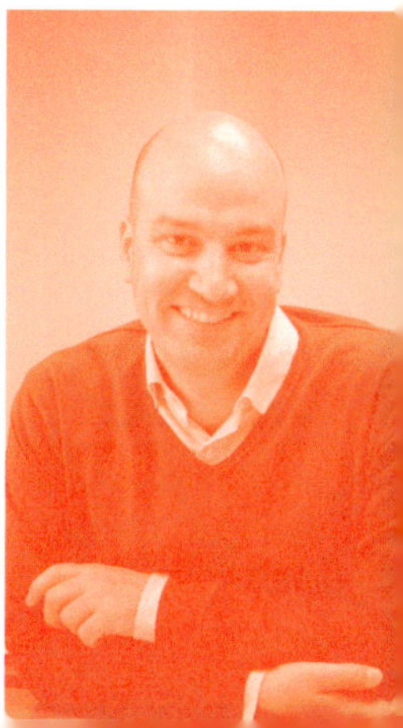

Gastritis - New Approaches and Treatments
http://dx.doi.org/10.5772/intechopen.77767
Edited by Bruna Maria Roesler

Contributors
Hirofumi Shimomura, Kiyofumi Wanibuchi, Hisashi Masui, Takashi Takahashi, Balaji Ommurugan, Vanishree Rao, Xiaomei Wang, Huangan Wu, Guang Ji, Mila Dimitrova Kovacheva-Slavova, Todor Asenov Angelov, Hristo Ilianov Iliev, Borislav Vladimirov, Hristo Yankov Valkov, Isidro Favian Bayas-Morejón, Rosa Angélica Tigre-León, Edison Riveliño Ramón-Curay, Darwin Alberto Nuñez-Torres

First published in London, United Kingdom, 2019 by IntechOpen
IntechOpen is the global imprint of INTECHOPEN LIMITED, registered in England and Wales, registration number: 11086078, 7th floor, 10 Lower Thames Street, London, EC3R 6AF, United Kingdom
Printed in Croatia

British Library Cataloguing-in-Publication Data
A catalogue record for this book is available from the British Library

Additional hard and PDF copies can be obtained from orders@intechopen.com

Gastritis - New Approaches and Treatments
Edited by Bruna Maria Roesler
p. cm.
Print ISBN 978-1-78984-664-5
Online ISBN 978-1-78984-665-2
eBook (PDF) ISBN 978-1-83968-009-0

For EU product safety concerns:
IN TECH d.o.o., Prolaz Marije Krucifikse Kozulić 3, 51000 Rijeka, Croatia, info@intechopen.com or visit our website at intechopen.com.

Meet the editor

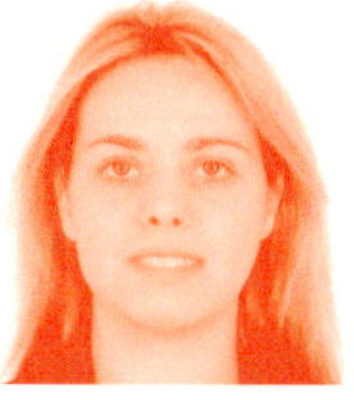

Dr. Bruna Maria Roesler is a pharmacist biochemist and holds a Master's degree in Pharmacology and a Doctoral degree in Basic Sciences—Internal Medicine from the State University of Campinas (Campinas, SP, Brazil) where she has identified the principal genotypes of *Helicobacter pylori* strains in patients with chronic gastritis, peptic ulcer disease, and gastric cancer (early and advanced stages) through molecular biology techniques. She has published her work in several peer-reviewed journals and given oral and poster presentations at various congresses. Her research also includes the etiology, epidemiology, and physiopathology of gastrointestinal diseases. She has also participated in studies that reported the possible relationship between *H. pylori* and idiopathic thrombocytopenic purpura, as well as between *H. pylori* and liver diseases.

Contents

Preface

This edited volume is a collection of reviewed and relevant research chapters concerning developments within the gastritis—new approaches and treatments field of study. The book includes scholarly contributions by various authors and is edited by a group of experts pertinent to gastritis, gastric carcinogenesis, and new approaches in diagnoses and treatments. Each contribution comes as a separate chapter complete in itself but directly related to the book's topics and objectives.

The book is divided into three sections: *Helicobacter pylori*: *General Comments*, *Diversity of Treatments for H. pylori Infection Worldwide*, and *Autoimmune Gastritis*.

The section *Helicobacter pylori*: *General Comments* includes chapters dealing with *Helicobacter pylori* Infection and *Helicobacter pylori*: A Pathogen of Ample Risk to Health.

The following section, *Diversity of Treatments for H. pylori Infection Worldwide*, includes Development of a Novel Antibacterial Medicine that Targets a Characteristic Lipid of the Cell Membranes of Helicobacter pylori, Pharmacotherapy of Peptic Ulcer Disease and Latest Research, and Gastritis Treated by Chinese Medicine.

Current View on Autoimmune Gastritis is included in the last section of this book, *Autoimmune Gastritis*.

The target audience comprises scholars and specialists in the field.

IntechOpen

Section 1

Helicobacter pylori: General Comments

Chapter 1

Helicobacter pylori Infection

Todor Asenov Angelov, Mila Dimitrova Kovacheva-Slavova, Hristo Ilianov Iliev, Hristo Yankov Valkov and Borislav Georgiev Vladimirov

Abstract

Helicobacter pylori (*H. pylori*) is a Gram-negative spiral bacterium commonly found in the stomach. Major part of the world's population is infected with *H. pylori* and is at increased risk of severe gastritis, peptic ulcer disease, and gastric cancer. Most studied virulence factors of the bacterium are the cytotoxin-associated gene (CagA) and the vacuolating cytotoxin A (VacA). The *H. pylori* infection is diagnosed by invasive (histological examination, culture, and rapid urease test, which require endoscopy and biopsy) and noninvasive methods (serology, urea breath test, and stool antigen test). *H. pylori* eradication is preferred for a long-term prevention of complications. Current treatments consist of antibiotics and adequate PPI dose and can be divided into two strands—with or without bismuth. Achieving an eradication rate of >90% is an indicator for effective treatment. Due to the increasing levels of antibiotic resistance, the standard triple therapy is largely replaced with a quadruple therapy, especially in countries with high resistance rates. Antimicrobial susceptibility testing should be performed after the second-line treatment failure, leading to an individualized patient treatment. Clear explanations and patients' compliance are of great importance for a better outcome.

Keywords: *Helicobacter pylori*, virulence factors, diagnostic methods, treatment

1. Introduction

In the early 1980s, *Helicobacter pylori* (*H. pylori*) was discovered by Barry Marshall and Robin Warren. They reported its presence on mucosal tissue from the stomach of patients with gastritis and peptic ulcers [1]. Today, it is known that more than half of Earth's population is infected with this Gram-negative spiral bacterium. In most cases, the infection is completely asymptomatic, but it is far from harmless as 10–15% of those infected will develop peptic ulcer disease or gastric cancer [2]. The type and severity of the disease depends on several factors, as characteristics of the colonizing strain, host immune response, smoking, high-salt diet, and presence of other concurrent infections [3].

H. pylori strains from different geographical areas show clear phylogeographic features. The bacterium follows the human migration and has co-evolved with humans for over at least 60,000 years [4]. The fecal-oral and oral-oral routes of transmission are most common, with close person-to-person contact required. Strains of *H. pylori* are usually isolated from gastric biopsy tissue specimens, but the bacterium can be recovered also from saliva, gastric reflux fluid, diarrhea, and vomitus. Isolation and transmission from contaminated water supplies and farm animals has also been reported [5].

H. pylori is "special" in many ways as it possesses several important enzymes that enable its survival in the hostile acidic environment. Such an enzyme is the urease, which breaks down the urea to ammonia and carbon dioxide, hence neutralizing the hydrochloric acid. Moreover, *H. pylori* avoids clearance with the gastric emptying with a number of adhesion molecules and its 4–6 flagella. Important virulence factors are the cytotoxin-associated gene A (CagA) and the vacuolating cytotoxin A (VacA).

Even though *H. pylori* colonization is usually asymptomatic, it leads to chronic active gastritis in most patients and is associated with a number of other gastroduodenal diseases, including gastric and duodenal ulcer disease, distal gastric adenocarcinoma, primary gastric mucosal-associated lymphoid tissue (MALT) lymphoma, dyspepsia, atrophic gastritis, iron deficiency anemia, and idiopathic thrombocytopenic purpura.

This is why *H. pylori* eradication is preferred for a long-term prevention of the above-mentioned complications. Current *H. pylori* treatment consists of antibiotics and adequate PPI dose and can be divided into two strands—with or without bismuth. Achievement of an eradication rate >90% is an indicator for effective treatment [6].

2. *H. pylori* virulence factors

H. pylori strains are more virulent and are associated with more severe gastric mucosal damages when there is a cytotoxin-associated gene pathogenicity island (cag PAI) in their genome. The cag PAI region contains ~30 genes encoding a type IV secretion system (T4SS) as well as cytotoxin-associated gene A (CagA). The CagA is delivered into host gastric epithelial cells via T4SS. Inside the cells, CagA undergoes tyrosine phosphorylation at the Glu-Pro-Ile-Tyr-Al (EPIYA) motifs by Src kinases. There is a higher risk for gastric cancer development in chronic infection with *H. pylori* cagA-positive strains. Carcinogenesis requires two major events. One is inactivation of tumor suppressor, and the other is the activation of oncoprotein. *H. pylori* CagA interacts with both of them and successfully disturbs their functions [7].

Vacuolating Cytotoxin (VacA) is also a major virulence factor present in almost all strains, and is highly polymorphic. VacA affects the cells with the induction of vacuole formation, mitochondrial dysfunction, modulation of signal transduction pathways, inhibition of T cell proliferation, and production of inflammatory cytokines. To favor its action, VacA binds to receptors such as receptor protein tyrosine phosphatases (RPTPα and RPTPβ), low-density lipoprotein receptor-related protein-1 (LRP1), fibronectin, CD18, and sphingomyelin. RPTPβ promote to ulceration and LRP1 is involved in the induction of autophagy. There is an interaction between cagA and VacA molecules, which is associated with the pathogenesis of gastric diseases. Therefore, further research on VacA may increase the knowledge of its role in the development of gastric disorders in *H. pylori* infection [7].

H. pylori expresses several major adhesins including BabA, SabA, LabA, OipA, and AlpAB. A closer association of the bacteria with the epithelium is thought to be mediated by them. They also increase the inflammation and damage of gastric mucosa by enhanced exposure to other virulence factors.

Duodenal ulcer-promoting gene A, dupA, is present in the tfs4 gene cluster and also the presence of the iceA1 allele of iceA is associated with increased risk for duodenal ulcer disease.

3. *Helicobacter pylori*-associated diseases

3.1 Dyspepsia

According to Rome III, functional dyspepsia (FD) is a symptomatic dyspepsia in the absence of structural or biochemical explanation after appropriate investigation [8]. There are gastrointestinal symptoms that are associated with chronic dyspepsia as epigastric pain, epigastric burning, uncomfortable postprandial fullness, and early satiation.

FD is one of the most common gastrointestinal diseases which affects the quality of life. Chronic dyspepsia symptoms, which are thought to be caused by *H. pylori* infection, are decided to be separated from FD and defined as *H. pylori*-associated dyspepsia (HpD) in the Kyoto Global Consensus Conference held on January 30–February 1, 2014 [9]. In this meeting, patients who remain symptom free 12 months after eradication are considered to be cases of HpD, while patients who continue to experience dyspepsia even after *H. pylori* eradication will be considered as FD [10].

The evidence of the association between *H. pylori* infection and dyspepsia has been increasing. However, it is still unknown why most of individuals with *H. pylori* infection have no symptoms, while some of them have chronic dyspepsia symptoms. Recent meta-analysis of 103 reports containing 312,415 individuals showed that the prevalence of uninvestigated dyspepsia was higher in *H. pylori*-positive individuals (OR 1.18; 95% CI 1.04–1.33) [11]. There is evidence of a small but statistically significant benefit in eradicating *H. pylori* in *H. pylori*-positive dyspepsia. Therefore, the eradication therapy is recommended as first-line therapy for *H. pylori*-positive dyspepsia. Zhao et al. reviewed 14 randomized controlled trials which contained information on the long-term (12 months or more) effects of *H. pylori* eradication on dyspeptic symptoms, and a sub-group analysis on geographical regions was conducted [12].

3.2 Gastritis

H. pylori swims through the layers of protective mucus of the gastric mucosa to avoid damage from gastric acid and digestive enzymes. The bacterium is able to interact with the mucins via major adhesins the blood group antigen-binding adhesin (BabA), sialic acid-binding adhesin (SabA), and the lacdiNAc-specific adhesin, LabA [13–15].

H. pylori activates inflammatory gene when the bacterium reach to gastric epithelial cells. This is possible due to interaction with Toll-like receptor 2 and NOD1 [16], and inflammasomes [17, 18]. Inflammatory signaling in gastric epithelial cells is activated by a number of different mechanisms, resulting in the secretion of cytokines and chemokines, including interleukin-8 (IL-8), IL-1b, tumor necrosis factor alpha (TNFa), IL-6, IL-12, CCL2-5, CCL20, and CXCL1-3 [19]. The chemokines leads to the accumulation of neutrophils, macrophages, mast cells, dendritic cells (DCs), innate lymphoid cells, and lymphocytes—gastritis [4].

Neutrophils, macrophages, and NK cells contribute to gastritis via the secretion of inflammatory and tissue-damaging factors including reactive oxygen and nitrogen species (ROS and RNS) [20], perforin, and granzymes [21]. However, DCs are semi-mature and tolerogenic in *H. pylori*-infected gastric mucosa that stimulate the development of regulatory T cells (Tregs), which suppress inflammation [22].

It has recently been shown that retinoic acid (RA) is produced by human gastric epithelial cells and DCs regulates the level of inflammation. More intense inflammation and mucosal damage have been observed during *H. pylori* infection, because of reduction in RA [23]. Autoreactive antibodies against molecules, such as the parietal cell H^+ and K^+-ATPase, frequently induce the molecular mimicry of *H. pylori*. These antibodies may enhance inflammation and damage in the stomach [24]. In addition, the cytokines interferon-gamma (IFNc) and TNFa, secreted by Th1 cells, stimulate macrophages to secrete further pro-inflammatory factors. IL-17A, IL-17F, IL-21, and IL-22, secreted by Th17 cells, also stimulate the expression of ROS, RNS, and chemokines, leading to further inflammation and neutrophil recruitment [25].

All of the above makes it clear that the hosts' immune response is one of the major factors involved in the *H. pylori* infection pathogenesis. Thus, cytokines and other chemokines, prostaglandins, and their metabolites, as products of the innate response may be involved in the etiology of *H. pylori*-related diseases.

3.3 Peptic ulcer disease

Around 95% of duodenal ulcers and around 70% of gastric ulcers are *H. pylori* infection related [26, 27]. Hemorrhage or perforation are relatively common complications and are associated with a significant mortality.

H. pylori infection leads to destruction of delta cells by chronic inflammation of the antrum. This leads to a reduction in the level of somatostatin secretion and therefore impaired inhibition of gastrin production by the G cells, causing hypergastrinemia. The elevated gastrin levels overstimulate the acid-producing parietal cells of the undamaged corpus (in the case of antral-predominant gastritis) resulting in hyperchlorhydria. The increased gastric acid output can result in gastric metaplasia of the duodenal epithelium. This allows *H. pylori* to colonize it and cause inflammation, possibly leading to duodenal ulceration.

On the other hand, in patients with corpus-predominant atrophy or pangastritis, the acid output can be normal or reduced, explained by the loss of parietal cells. A state of hypochlorhydria is established, despite increased gastrin production from the *H. pylori*-infected antrum, preventing development of duodenal ulcers. Gastric ulcers develop due to inflammation and damage to the gastric mucosa. Premalignant lesions and gastric adenocarcinoma may also develop [4, 28].

In those with reduced numbers of Tregs in their gastric mucosa, peptic ulceration is more frequently found thus impaired capacity to control the inflammation [19, 29]. The inflammation and damage are enhanced by gastric Th1 and Th17 cells inducing epithelial cells to express higher levels of MHC class II and activation of mitogen-activated protein (MAP) kinases and transcription factors AP-1 and NF-jB [30].

3.4 Gastric adenocarcinoma

There are approximately 100,000 new cases of gastric cancer each year [31]. A majority of cases are registered in developing countries, half of them occurring in Eastern Asia. It is the fifth most common malignancy worldwide and the third most common cause of cancer-related death diagnosed usually at a late stage [32].

Depending on the location the gastric cancer can be divided into two subtypes:

- Cardia—arising from epithelial cells at the gastroesophageal junction.
- Non-cardia—arising from the distal stomach.

Cardia gastric cancers are thought to be mostly unrelated to *H. pylori* infection and have similar risk factors to those for esophageal adenocarcinoma and Barrett's esophagus [30]. Up to 89% of cases of non-cardia gastric cancer is attributed to the infection with *H. pylori*. The risk of gastric cancer development for an infected individual is 1–2% [33].

The gastric cancer is classified histologically as two types [34]:

- intestinal—usually exophytic, often ulcerating, and are associated with intestinal metaplasia of the stomach and are more common in proximal (fundus) location.

- diffuse-type—poorly differentiated infiltrating lesions, which lead to the thickening of the stomach (linitis plastica) and predominate in younger patients.

Patients with intestinal-type tumors appear to have a better prognosis than those with diffuse-type.

Chronic gastritis caused by *H. pylori* infection after several decades, leads to gastric gland atrophy, intestinal metaplasia, dysplasia, and finally adenocarcinoma. *H. pylori* eradication therapy reduces the incidence of atrophic gastritis, but the risk of gastric cancer development is reduced only if the eradication is administered prior to pre-malignant changes [35]. ROS/RNS-mediated DNA damage, the silencing of tumor suppressor genes via DNA methylation, histone epigenetic modifications, and epithelial-mesenchymal transition are associated with gastric carcinogenesis [36].

Genetically determined high expression of pro-inflammatory cytokines (IL-6, IL-8, TNFa, IL-1b), low expression of anti-inflammatory cytokines (IL-10, TGFb), or enhanced responsiveness to bacterial components (Toll-like receptors 1, 2, 4, 5, and 9) are associated with a higher risk of gastric adenocarcinoma [37, 38]. In the future, identification of molecular profiles for gastric cancer subtypes will lead to more personalized clinical management, therapeutic targets and biomarkers for screening, prognosis, prediction of response to treatment, and monitoring of gastric cancer progression [39].

3.5 MALT lymphoma

Almost all patients with gastric MALT lymphoma have an active *H. pylori* infection with frequency of approximately 0.8 per 100,000 per year. Around 10% of cases are thought to be independent of *H. pylori*, but may be due to perhaps gastric non-pylori Helicobacters or undiagnosed *H. pylori* infection. Formation of lymphoid follicles in the gastric mucosa is induced by *H. pylori*-mediated inflammation, which is not present in the uninfected stomach [40]. Chronic inflammation and continuous antigenic stimulation lead to uncontrolled expansion of marginal zone B cells in these lymphoid follicles [41]. The tumor cells are commonly localized in the gastric mucosa and often remain to this site. However, in approximately 40% of cases, spreading to regional lymph nodes and more distant mucosal sites occurs. In around half of gastric lymphoma, low-grade MALT lymphomas may transform into more aggressive diffuse large B cell lymphomas (DLBCL), which have a considerably worse prognosis [41]. After *H. pylori* eradication treatment, there is a regression of the low-grade B cell MALT lymphomas. In one-quarter of cases a chromosomal translocation t(11; 18) is found. This is the most common genetic aberration in gastric MALT lymphoma. The non-responsiveness of gastric MALT lymphoma to *H. pylori* eradication therapy is also predicted by the presence of t(11; 18) [42]. Fusion between the activator protein-12 (AP-12) and MALT-1 genes lead to this chromosomal breakage and translocation. The product of this fusion stimulates activation of the transcription factor NF-jB, which regulates the expression of anti-apoptotic genes and cell survival [41]. Mutations in immunoglobulin heavy chain variable region (IGHV) genes are also frequently present [43]. There is growing evidence that host genetic factors play an important role in developing gastric MALT lymphoma.

4. Diagnosis

Diagnosis of *H. pylori* infection can be done with noninvasive methods—serology, urea breath test (UBT), stool antigen test (SAT)—and invasive methods—histology, culture, PCR, rapid urease test (RUT). Only locally validated tests should be used. PPIs have an anti-*H. pylori* activity and decrease the load of *H. pylori* leading to false-negative results on urease test, UBT, and SAT [44]. H2 receptor antagonists have been shown to have minimal effect on the sensitivity of UBT, and antacids do not impair the sensitivity of UBT or SAT. H2-blockers do not have anti-*H. pylori* activity [45–47]. In contrast, the antibacterial activity of antibiotics and bismuth compounds necessitate their discontinuation for 4 weeks to allow an increase of a detectable bacterial load.

From the noninvasive methods, 13C-UBT is the best approach to the diagnosis of *H. pylori* infection, with high sensitivity and specificity [48–50]. It cannot be used in children and pregnant women, because it exposes the patients to radiation [51]. SAT may be less acceptable in some societies, but has a high sensitivity and specificity [6]. Under certain clinical circumstances, it leads to a low bacterial load in the stomach and to a decreased sensitivity of all diagnostic methods except serology. These clinical situations include GI bleeding, atrophic gastritis, gastric MALT lymphoma, and gastric carcinoma. Because serology is able to detect past infection with *H. pylori*, it should not be used as a method to monitor effectiveness of eradication.

In clinical practice, when there is an indication for endoscopy, and there is no contraindication for biopsy, the rapid urease test (RUT) is recommended as a first-line diagnostic test [6]. The sensitivity of biopsy urease tests is approximately 90%, and specificity is in the range of 95–100% [52]. It has been shown that the best biopsy sites for detection of *H. pylori* and assessment of atrophy are the lesser and greater curvature of the mid antrum, and the middle gastric body at the lesser and greater curvature [53]. This is supported by the updated Sydney System [54]. A maximum approach for gastric biopsies includes the incisura region at the lesser curvature. In the case of detection of gastric polyps, ulcerations, and suspicious focal lesions, further biopsies are necessary.

Most cases of *H. pylori* infection can be diagnosed from gastric biopsies using histochemical staining alone. In cases of chronic (active) gastritis in which *H. pylori* is not detected by histochemistry, immunohistochemical testing of *H. pylori* can be used as an accessory test. In the case of normal histology, no immunohistochemical staining should be performed [6].

The value of culture is primarily to perform AST for clarithromycin, levofloxacin, metronidazole, rifamycin, and eventually, amoxicillin and tetracycline. Several studies, using tailored treatments based on *H. pylori* susceptibility to antibiotics in comparison with standard empirical triple therapy, have shown a better eradication rate and may be cost-effective [55, 56].

A panel of serological tests (GastroPanel), including serum Pg (PgI and PgII), gastrin 17 (G-17), and anti-*H. pylori* antibodies, has recently been proposed as "serological biopsy" in dyspeptic patients [57, 58]. In populations with a low prevalence of atrophic gastritis, the negative predictive value of the GastroPanel in identifying atrophic gastritis is as high as 97% (95% CI 95–99%) [59].

In the post-treatment evaluation, UBT is a valid and reliable test in the assessment of *H. pylori* eradication [60]. SAT can be used as an alternative [61]. Testing to prove eradication should be performed at least 4–8 weeks after completion of *H. pylori* therapy. PPI should be discontinued for at least 2 weeks [48, 61–63].

5. Treatment

Recommended treatment regimens [64]:

Clarithromycin triple—PPI (standard or double dose twice daily) + clarithromycin (500 mg twice daily) + amoxicillin (1 g twice daily) **OR** metronidazole (500 mg three times daily) for 14 days.

Bismuth quadruple—PPI (standard dose twice daily) + bismuth subcitrate (120–300 mg 4 times daily) or subsalicylate (300 mg 4 times daily) + tetracycline (500 mg 4 times daily) + metronidazole (250 mg 4 times daily or 500 mg 3–4 times daily) for 10–14 days.

Concomitant—PPI (standard dose twice daily) + clarithromycin (500 mg twice daily) + amoxicillin (1 g twice daily) + nitroimidazole (500 mg twice daily).

Suggested [64]:

Sequential—PPI (standard dose twice daily) + amoxicillin (1 g twice daily) for 5–7 days **then** PPI + clarithromycin (500 mg twice daily) + nitroimidazole5 (500 mg twice daily) for 5–7 days.

Hybrid—PPI (standard dose twice daily) + amoxicillin (1 g twice daily) for 7 days **then** PPI + amoxicillin + clarithromycin (500 mg twice daily) + nitroimidazole (500 mg twice daily) 7 days.

Levofloxacin triple—PPI (standard dose twice daily) + levofloxacin (500 mg daily) + amoxicillin (1 g twice daily) for 14 days.

Levofloxacin sequential—PPI (standard or double dose twice daily) + amoxicillin (1 g twice daily) for 5–7 days **then** PPI + levofloxacin (500 mg daily) + nitroimidazole5 (500 mg twice daily) for 5–7 days.

LOAD—Levofloxacin (250 mg daily) + omeprazole (double dose daily) + nitazoxanide (500 mg twice daily) + doxycycline (100 mg daily) for 7–10 days.

Eradication rates of *H. pylori* have been declining, because of the increasing resistance rates to antibiotics worldwide [65]. Such evidence comes from studies in Europe, Japan, Korea, China, Iran, Greece, Bulgaria, and others [66–71]. Clarithromycin resistance rates have now reached ~30% in Italy and Japan, ~40% in Turkey, and ~50% in China, although rates in Sweden and Taiwan were ~15%. The standard triple therapy is less effective nowadays, because of a number of reasons such as lower compliance, high gastric acidity, high bacterial load, and bacterial strains, but mainly due to the increase in *H. pylori* resistance to clarithromycin. *H. pylori* is now an inconstantly susceptible bacterium (10–50% resistant) except in Northern Europe. The choice of therapy should be based on the frequency of metronidazole and dual clarithromycin and metronidazole resistance. If metronidazole resistance is almost negligible (e.g., Japan), replacing clarithromycin for metronidazole in triple therapy (i.e., PPI-metronidazole-amoxicillin) shows excellent cure rates [72]. However, metronidazole resistance can be partially overcome by increasing the dose, frequency, and duration of the antibiotic.

All non-BQTs will be less effective in regions with dual resistance to clarithromycin and metronidazole >15% [73]. Non-bismuth quadruple concomitant therapy, prescribed for 14 days, can be an effective alternative in regions with high clarithromycin resistance (15–40%) but low to intermediate metronidazole resistance (<40%) [74]. Bismuth-containing quadruple therapies are the treatment of choice when we have high (>15%) dual clarithromycin and metronidazole resistance. Ideally, clarithromycin should be avoided and a combination of alternative antibiotics. If bismuth is not available in high dual clarithromycin and metronidazole resistance areas, levofloxacin [75], rifabutin [76], and high dose dual (PPI + amoxicillin) [77] treatments can be considered. Quadruple therapy with a PPI, bismuth, and a combination of two antibiotics, among furazolidone, tetracycline, metronidazole, and amoxicillin, has been successfully tested (>90% cure rates) against *H. pylori* strains resistant to metronidazole, fluoroquinolones, and clarithromycin [78] and now is the recommended first-line treatment [79]. BQT should be considered effective provided the doses are sufficient and the duration should be extended to 14 days, unless 10 day therapies are proven effective locally [80, 81]. The combination of PPI, bismuth, metronidazole, and tetracycline lasting 10–14 days achieved ≥85% eradication rate, even in areas with a high prevalence of metronidazole resistance [82–84].

Sequential therapy is more complex and requires switching of antibiotic drugs during the treatment course, which can confuse the patients. Concomitant therapy (PPI, amoxicillin, clarithromycin, and a nitroimidazole administered concurrently) is easier and similar to standard triple therapy and should be the preferred non-bismuth quadruple therapy. Sequential therapy achieves lower cure rates compared to concomitant therapy against clarithromycin-resistant strains [85, 86]. All non-BQTs (concomitant, hybrid, triple, and sequential) lead to excellent cure rates against susceptible *H. pylori* strains, but the cure rate will always be <90% when the rate of dual resistant strains is >5, >9, or >15%, respectively [73].

Response to PPI is individual and determined by cytochrome 2C19 and MDR polymorphisms. Caucasian subjects show a higher prevalence of high metabolizers (56–81%) compared to Asian [74]. Esomeprazole and rabeprazole provide better overall *H. pylori* eradication rates, especially esomeprazole 40 mg twice daily, whereas rabeprazole 10 and 20 mg twice daily [87–92]. By raising pH, *H. pylori* enters the replicative state and become susceptible to amoxicillin and clarithromycin [93].

For second-line treatment, after failure of PPI-clarithromycin-amoxicillin triple therapy, a bismuth-containing quadruple therapy or a fluoroquinolone-containing triple or quadruple therapy are recommended [94]. In theory, any treatment could be used after failure of BQT, including repeating the same BQT with longer duration and high metronidazole dosage. However, treatment that has already failed seems wiser never to be repeated. Bismuth therapies are usually proposed as first-line treatments for areas of high clarithromycin resistance and using a clarithromycin-containing treatment as second-line therapy after failure of a BQT does not seem to be practical. That is why Levofloxacin-based triple therapy, that is known to be effective as second-line therapy after clarithromycin-containing therapy, should also be recommended after failure of a bismuth-containing quadruple regimen [95, 96]. The incidence of side effects are lower with levofloxacin-containing triple therapy than with bismuth-containing quadruple therapy [97]. A sub-group analysis showed similar eradication rates with 500 and 1000 mg) of levofloxacin [97]. However, the efficacy of levofloxacin-based regimens may be affected by an increased prevalence of levofloxacin resistance [98]. Therefore, 14-day bismuth quadruple therapy is a valid second-line treatment for *H. pylori* eradication, especially in areas with high fluoroquinolones resistance. Combining bismuth and levofloxacin in a 14-day quadruple therapy is an effective (≥90% cure rate), simple, and safe second-line strategy in patients [99]. Bismuth overcomes clarithromycin and levofloxacin resistance, because of the synergistic effect with antibiotics [100, 101]. Therefore, the levofloxacin/bismuth-containing quadruple therapy constitutes an encouraging second-line strategy not only in patients failing previous standard triple therapy, but also in non-bismuth quadruple “sequential” or “concomitant” treatments.

After failure of the first-line treatment (clarithromycin based) and second-line treatment (with bismuth-containing quadruple regimen), it is recommended to use the fluoroquinolone-containing regimen as a rescue therapy. After failure of the first-line treatment (triple or non-bismuth quadruple) and second-line treatment (fluoroquinolone-containing therapy), it is recommended to use the bismuth-based quadruple therapy. Furthermore, BQT is not influenced by clarithromycin and fluoroquinolone resistance [102]. However, if a second-line treatment fails, culture with susceptibility testing (AST) or molecular determination of genotype resistance is recommended. Susceptibility-guided triple therapies proved more effective than empirical triple therapies in first-line treatment [55, 103].

6. *Helicobacter pylori* and extragastric diseases

Chronic infection with *H. pylori* may be favorable for certain gastroesophageal diseases, asthma, and other allergic disease manifestations and inflammatory bowel diseases (IBD). The beneficial role of *H. pylori* in GERD, Barrett's esophagus (BE), and esophageal adenocarcinoma (EA) requires further clinical and experimental confirmation.

The reflux of gastric contents and the failure of the esophagus to clear by peristaltic contractions lead to GERD. The severity of the disease depends strongly on the pH of the refluxed gastric juice [104, 105]. Chronic GERDs most likely to cause BE—replacement of the stratified squamous epithelium with a metaplastic columnar epithelium. The inflammation caused by chronic acid exposure appear to promote the development of EA from BE [106]. Patients subjected to endoscopy for any indications have the prevalence of BE, which is approximately 1–2% up to 5–15% in patients with GERD symptoms. Patients with BE have a 30- to 125-fold higher risk for developing EA, in comparison with the general population [107].

In 2013, Rubenstein et al. found an inverse correlation of *H. pylori* with erosive esophagitis, especially in patients harboring CagA-positive strains [108]. This evidence was further supported by Korean and Japanese studies, in which *H. pylori* could be negatively linked with the risk and severity of erosive esophagitis [109, 110].

In 2012, Fischbach et al. documented a decreased risk of EA predominantly in patients infected with CagA-positive *H. pylori* strains and recently confirmed a negative association of *H. pylori* with the risk of BE [41, 111]. Nie et al. also found that CagA-positive *H. pylori* strains were associated with a decreased risk of EA in all populations, irrespective of geographical location [112].

Numerous studies have addressed whether *H. pylori* eradication promotes the development of GERD or associated diseases. However, recent studies have failed to corroborate an important clinical impact on GERD of *H. pylori* eradication.

Inflammatory bowel diseases (IBDs) are chronic relapsing disorders of increasing incidence and two main forms—Crohn's disease and ulcerative colitis. Intestinal inflammation and epithelial injury are characterized for the diseases. In Crohn's disease, inflammation is discontinuous and can affect any part of the gastrointestinal tract and all layers of the bowel wall. In contrast, ulcerative colitis expands continuously from the rectum and affect the superficial layer of the mucosa. Modern hygienic practices and diet have been proposed to account for the increasing incidence of IBD in Western societies associated with changes in the human microbiota composition [113]. A correlation between *H. pylori* infection and IBD has long been suspected by gastroenterologists. There is a lower prevalence of *H. pylori* in IBD patients confirmed by studies, in which active *H. pylori* infection was detected by urea breath test rather than serum IgG or IgA [114–116]. A strong negative association between *H. pylori* colonization and IBD is presented in all meta-analyses and almost all original articles covering the topic [117–119].

7. *H. pylori* and the human microbiota

H. pylori is its best-known component of the stomach microbiota. In healthy conditions the main representatives of gastric microbiota are Streptococcus, Proteobacteria, Firmicutes, Bacteroidetes, and Actinobacteria [120–124]. The exact composition of a healthy gastric microbiota remains uncharacterized. The interaction between the normal microbiota and *H. pylori* has not yet been fully defined. There is some evidence suggesting a predominance of *H. pylori* over other microbes

[120]. Non-*H. pylori Helicobacter* species can cause gastritis, peptic ulcer disease, gastric cancer, and gastric mucosa-associated lymphoid tissue lymphoma [125–130].

H. pylori eradication therapy can impair the healthy gut microbiota. The most relevant shifts involved are, respectively, *Bacteroides*, *Bifidobacterium*, *Clostridium*, *Enterobacteriaceae*, and *Lactobacillus* [131]. The most common GI side effects correlated with antibiotic therapy include diarrhea, nausea, vomiting, bloating, and abdominal pain [132]. Antibiotic administration is the main risk factor for the development of *C. difficile* infection [133]. There is insufficient evidence on the effect of different eradication regimens and long-lasting impact of *H. pylori* eradication on the composition of gut microbiota. There are encouraging results, that probiotic supplementation reduce the side effects of eradication [134–144]. Certain probiotics stains may have a better beneficial effect. There are evidence that *Saccharomyces boulardii* decreases the risk and overall adverse effects (RR 0.44, 95% CI 0.31 to 0.64) [145]. A number of meta-analyses of RCTs show a positive result that probiotics has the capacity to increase the efficacy of *H. pylori* eradication therapies [134–144]. Despite these encouraging data, probiotics appear to increase the *H. pylori* eradication rate not by direct effects on *H. pylori*, but with reducing the side effects related to the therapy.

8. Conclusion

Helicobacter pylori has been part of the human population and migration since ancient times. Infection with the bacterium is an extremely significant disease and can lead to severe consequences for infected individuals. Treatment and the rising bacterial resistance are challenges that we encounter in everyday practice, according to the latest guidelines recommendations. We hope that in the future our knowledge will expand and we will be ready to present new approaches for *H. pylori* management, because the bacterium will undoubtedly continue to be part of our microbiome.

Acknowledgments

The publication of this work was supported by KRKA.

Author details

Todor Asenov Angelov[1*], Mila Dimitrova Kovacheva-Slavova[1], Hristo Ilianov Iliev[2], Hristo Yankov Valkov [1] and Borislav Georgiev Vladimirov[1]

1 Department of Gastroenterology, University Hospital "Tsaritsa Ioanna-ISUL" Medical University of Sofia, Sofia, Bulgaria

2 Medical University of Sofia, Sofia, Bulgaria

*Address all correspondence to: totodari@gmail.com

References

[1] Marshall BJ, Warren JR. Unidentified curved bacilli in the stomach of patients with gastritis and peptic ulceration. Lancet. 1984;**1**(8390):1311-1315

[2] Torre LA, Bray F, Siegel RL, Ferlay J, Lortet-Tieulent J, Jemal A. Global cancer statistics, 2012. CA: A Cancer Journal for Clinicians. 2015;**65**(2):87-108. DOI: 10.3322/caac.21262

[3] Amieva M, Peek RM Jr. Pathobiology of *Helicobacter pylori*-induced gastric cancer. Gastroenterology. 2016;**150**(1): 64-78. DOI: 10.1053/j.gastro.2015.09.004

[4] Atherton JC, Blaser MJ. Coadaptation of *Helicobacter pylori* and humans: Ancient history, modern implications. The Journal of Clinical Investigation. 2009;**119**(9):2475-2487. DOI: 10.1172/JCI38605

[5] Breckan RK, Paulssen EJ, Asfeldt AM, Kvamme JM, Straume B, Florholmen J. The all-age prevalence of *Helicobacter pylori* infection and potential transmission routes. A population-based study. Helicobacter. 2016;**21**(6):586-595. DOI: 10.1111/hel.12316

[6] Malfertheiner P, Megraud F, O'Morain CA, Gisbert JP, Kuipers EJ, Axon AT, et al. Management of *Helicobacter pylori* infection—The Maastricht V/Florence Consensus Report. Gut. 2017;**66**(1):6-30. DOI: 10.1136/gutjnl-2016-312288

[7] Suzuki H, Warren R, Marshall B. *Helicobacter pylori*. Japan: Springer; 2016. DOI: 10.1007/978-4-431-55705-0. ISBN: 978-4-431-55704-3

[8] Tack J, Talley NJ, Camilleri M, Holtmann G, Hu P, Malagelada JR, et al., European Helicobacter and Microbiota Study Group and Consensus Panel. Functional gastroduodenal disorders. Gastroenterology. 2006;**130**(5):1466-1479. DOI: 10.1053/j.gastro.2005.11.059

[9] Sugano K, Tack J, Kuipers EJ, Graham DY, El-Omar EM, Miura S, et al. Kyoto global consensus report on *Helicobacter pylori* gastritis. Gut. 2015;**64**(9):1353-1367. DOI: 10.1136/gutjnl-2015-309252

[10] Miwa H, Kusano M, Arisawa T, Oshima T, Kato M, Joh T, et al. Evidence-based clinical practice guidelines for functional dyspepsia. Journal of Gastroenterology. 2015;**50**(2):125-139. DOI: 10.1007/ s00535-014-1022-3

[11] Ford AC, Marwaha A, Sood R, Moayyedi P. Global prevalence of, and risk factors for, uninvestigated dyspepsia: A meta-analysis. Gut. Jul 2015;**64**(7):1049-1057. DOI: 10.1136/gutjnl-2014-307843

[12] Zhao B, Zhao J, Cheng WF, Shi WJ, Liu W, Pan XL, et al. Efficacy of *Helicobacter pylori* eradication therapy on functional dyspepsia: A meta-analysis of randomized controlled studies with 12-month follow-up. Journal of Clinical Gastroenterology. 2014;**48**(3):241-247. DOI: 10.1097/MCG.0b013e31829f2e25

[13] Ilver D, Arnqvist A, Ogren J, Frick IM, Kersulyte D, Incecik ET, et al. *Helicobacter pylori* adhesin binding fucosylated histo-blood group antigens revealed by retagging. Science. 1998;**279**(5349):373-377

[14] Mahdavi J, Sonden B, Hurtig M, Olfat FO, Forsberg L, Roche N, et al. *Helicobacter pylori* SabA adhesin in persistent infection and chronic inflammation. Science. 2002;**297**(5581):573-578. DOI: 10.1126/science.1069076

[15] Rossez Y, Gosset P, Boneca IG, Magalhaes A, Ecobichon C, Reis CA, et al. The lacdiNAc-specific adhesin LabA mediates adhesion of *Helicobacter pylori* to human gastric mucosa.

The Journal of Infectious Diseases. 2014;**210**(8):1286-1295. DOI: 10.1093/infdis/jiu239

[16] Viala J, Chaput C, Boneca IG, Cardona A, Girardin SE, Moran AP, et al. Nod1 responds to peptidoglycan delivered by the *Helicobacter pylori* cag pathogenicity island. Nature Immunology. 2004;**5**(11):1166-1174

[17] Kim DJ, Park JH, Franchi L, Backert S, Núñez G. The Cag pathogenicity island and interaction between TLR2/NOD2 and NLRP3 regulate IL-1b production in *Helicobacter pylori* infected dendritic cells. European Journal of Immunology. 2013;**43**(10):2650-2658. DOI: 10.1002/eji.201243281

[18] Vanaja SK, Rathinam VA, Fitzgerald KA. Mechanisms of inflammasome activation: Recent advances and novel insights. Trends in Cell Biology. 2015;**25**(5):308-315. DOI: 10.1016/j.tcb.2014.12.009

[19] Cook KW, Letley DP, Ingram RJ, Staples E, Skjoldmose H, Atherton JC, et al. CCL20/CCR6-mediated migration of regulatory T cells to the *Helicobacter pylori*-infected human gastric mucosa. Gut. 2014;**63**(10):1550-1559. DOI: 10.1136/gutjnl-2013-306253

[20] Italiani P, Boraschi D. From monocytes to M1/M2 macrophages: Phenotypical vs. functional differentiation. Frontiers in Immunology. 2014;**5**:514. DOI: 10.3389/fimmu.2014.00514

[21] Yun CH, Lundgren A, Azem J, Sjoling A, Holmgren J, Svennerholm AM, et al. Natural killer cells and *Helicobacter pylori* infection: Bacterial antigens and interleukin-12 act synergistically to induce gamma interferon production. Infection and Immunity. 2005;**73**(3):1482-1490

[22] Rizzuti D, Ang M, Sokollik C, Wu T, Abdullah M, Greenfield L, et al. *Helicobacter pylori* inhibits dendritic cell maturation via interleukin-10-mediated activation of the signal transducer and activator of transcription 3 pathway. Journal of Innate Immunity. 2015;**7**(2):199-211. DOI: 10.1159/000368232

[23] Bimczok D, Kao JY, Zhang M, Cochrun S, Mannon P, Peter S, et al. Human gastric epithelial cells contribute to gastric immune regulation by providing retinoic acid to dendritic cells. Mucosal Immunology. May 2015;**8**(3):533-544. DOI: 10.1038/mi.2014.86

[24] Smyk DS, Koutsoumpas AL, Mytilinaiou MG, Rigopoulou EI, Sakkas LI, Bogdanos DP. *Helicobacter pylori* and autoimmune disease: Cause or bystander. World Journal of Gastroenterology. 2014;**20**(3):613-629. DOI: 10.3748/wjg.v20.i3.613

[25] Oertli M, Sundquist M, Hitzler I, Engler DB, Arnold IC, Reuter S, et al. DC-derived IL-18 drives Treg differentiation, murine *Helicobacter pylori*-specific immune tolerance, and asthma protection. The Journal of Clinical Investigation. 2012;**122**(3):1082-1096. DOI: 10.1172/JCI61029

[26] Ford AC, Gurusamy KS, Delaney B, Forman D, Moayyedi P. Eradication therapy for peptic ulcer disease in *Helicobacter pylori*-positive people. Cochrane Database of Systematic Reviews. 2016;**4**:CD003840. DOI: 10.1002/14651858.CD003840.pub5

[27] Malfertheiner P. The intriguing relationship of *Helicobacter pylori* infection and acid secretion in peptic ulcer disease and gastric cancer. Digestive Diseases. 2011;**29**(5):459-464. DOI: 10.1159/000332213

[28] Robinson K, Kenefeck R, Pidgeon EL, Shakib S, Patel S, Polson RJ, et al. *Helicobacter pylori*-induced peptic

ulcer disease is associated with inadequate regulatory T cell responses. Gut. 2008;**57**(10):1375-1385

[29] Zhou Y, Toh ML, Zrioual S, Miossec P. IL-17A versus IL-17F induced intracellular signal transduction pathways and modulation by IL-17RA and IL-17RC RNA interference in AGS gastric adenocarcinoma cells. Cytokine. 2007;**38**(3):157-164. DOI: 10.1016/j.cyto.2007.06.002

[30] Colquhoun A, Arnold M, Ferlay J, Goodman KJ, Forman D, Soerjomataram I. Global patterns of cardia and non-cardia gastric cancer incidence in 2012. Gut. 2015;**64**(12):1881-1888. DOI: 10.1136/gutjnl-2014-308915

[31] Herrero R, Park JY, Forman D. The fight against gastric cancer—The IARC Working Group report. Best Practice & Research. Clinical Gastroenterology. 2014;**28**(6):1107-1114. DOI: 10.1016/j.bpg.2014.10.003

[32] Plummer M, Franceschi S, Vignat J, Forman D, de Martel C. Global burden of gastric cancer attributable to *Helicobacter pylori*. International Journal of Cancer. 2015;**136**(2):487-490. DOI: 10.1002/ijc.28999

[33] Lauren P. The two histological main types of gastric carcinoma: Diffuse and so-called intestinal-type carcinoma. An attempt at a histo-clinical classification. Acta Pathologica et Microbiologica Scandinavica. 1965;**64**:31-49

[34] Malfertheiner P, Fry LC, Monkemuller K. Can gastric cancer be prevented by *Helicobacter pylori* eradication? Best Practice & Research. Clinical Gastroenterology. 2006;**20**(4):709-719. DOI: 10.1016/j.bpg.2006.04.005

[35] Na HK, Woo JH. *Helicobacter pylori* induces hypermethylation of CpG islands through upregulation of DNA methyltransferase: Possible involvement of reactive oxygen/nitrogen species. Journal of Cancer Prevention. 2014;**19**(4):259-264. DOI: 10.15430/JCP.2014.19.4.259

[36] Ramis IB, Vianna JS, Goncalves CV, von Groll A, Dellagostin OA, da Silva PE. Polymorphisms of the IL-6, IL-8 and IL-10 genes and the risk of gastric pathology in patients infected with *Helicobacter pylori*. Journal of Microbiology, Immunology, and Infection. 2015;**9**(12):1535-1547. DOI: 10.1016/j.jmii.2015.03.002

[37] El-Omar EM, Ng MT, Hold GL. Polymorphisms in toll-like receptor genes and risk of cancer. Oncogene. 2008;**27**(2):244-252

[38] Tegtmeyer N, Backert S. Molecular Pathogenesis and Signal Transduction by *Helicobacter pylori*. Part of Current Topics in Microbiology and Immunology. Cham, Switzerland: Springer International Publishing AG; 2017;**400**. DOI: 10.1007/978-3-319-50520-6. ISBN: 978-3-319-50519-0

[39] Genta RM, Hamner HW, Graham DY. Gastric lymphoid follicles in *Helicobacter pylori* infection: Frequency, distribution, and response to triple therapy. Human Pathology. 1993;**24**(6):577-583

[40] Du MQ, Atherton JC. Molecular subtyping of gastric MALT lymphomas: Implications for prognosis and management. Gut. 2006;**55**(6):886-893

[41] Fischbach W. Gastric MALT lymphoma—Update on diagnosis and treatment. Best Practice & Research. Clinical Gastroenterology. 2014;**28**(6):1069-1077. DOI: 10.1016/j.bpg.2014.09.006

[42] Zucca E, Bertoni F. The spectrum of MALT lymphoma at different sites: Biological and therapeutic relevance.

Blood. 2016;**127**(17):2082-2092. DOI: 10.1182/blood-2015-12-624304

[43] Gatta L, Vakil N, Ricci C, et al. Effect of proton pump inhibitors and antacid therapy on 13C urea breath tests and stool test for *Helicobacter pylori* infection. The American Journal of Gastroenterology. 2004;**99**:823-829

[44] Connor SJ, Ngu MC, Katelaris PH. The impact of short-term ranitidine use on the precision of the 13C-urea breath test in subjects infected with *Helicobacter pylori*. European Journal of Gastroenterology & Hepatology. 1999;**11**:1135-1138

[45] Savarino V, Tracci D, Dulbecco P, et al. Negative effect of ranitidine on the results of urea breath test for the diagnosis of *Helicobacter pylori*. The American Journal of Gastroenterology. 2001;**96**:348-352

[46] Dulbecco P, Gambaro C, Bilardi C, et al. Impact of long-term ranitidine and pantoprazole on accuracy of [13C] urea breath test. Digestive Diseases and Sciences. 2003;**48**:315-321

[47] Gisbert JP, Calvet X. *Helicobacter pylori* 'test-and-treat' strategy for management of dyspepsia: A comprehensive review. Clinical and Translational Gastroenterology. 2013;**4**:e32

[48] Gisbert JP, Pajares JM. Review article: 13C-urea breath test in the diagnosis of *Helicobacter pylori* infection—A critical review. Alimentary Pharmacology & Therapeutics. 2004;**20**:1001-1017

[49] Nocon M, Kuhlmann A, Leodolter A, et al. Efficacy and cost-effectiveness of the 13C-urea breath test as the primary diagnostic investigation for the detection of *Helicobacter pylori* infection compared to invasive and non-invasive diagnostic tests. GMS Health Technology Assessment. 2009;**5**:Doc14

[50] Ferwana M, Abdulmajeed I, Alhajiahmed A, et al. Accuracy of urea breath test in *Helicobacter pylori* infection: Meta-analysis. World Journal of Gastroenterology. 2015;**21**: 1305-1314

[51] Gisbert JP, de la Morena F, Abraira V. Accuracy of monoclonal stool antigen test for the diagnosis of *H. pylori* infection: A systematic review and meta-analysis. The American Journal of Gastroenterology. 2006;**101**:1921-1930

[52] El-Zimaity HM, Al-Assi MT, Genta RM, et al. Confirmation of successful therapy of *Helicobacter pylori* infection: Number and site of biopsies or a rapid urease test. The American Journal of Gastroenterology. 1995;**90**:1962-1964

[53] Satoh K, Kimura K, Taniguchi Y, et al. Biopsy sites suitable for the diagnosis of *Helicobacter pylori* infection and the assessment of the extent of atrophic gastritis. The American Journal of Gastroenterology. 1998;**93**:569-573

[54] Dixon MF, Genta RM, Yardley JH, et al. Classification and grading of gastritis. The updated Sydney System. International Workshop on the Histopathology of Gastritis, Houston 1994. The American Journal of Surgical Pathology. 1996;**20**:1161-1181

[55] Wenzhen Y, Yumin L, Quanlin G, et al. Is antimicrobial susceptibility testing necessary before first-line treatment for *Helicobacter pylori* infection? Meta-analysis of randomized controlled trials. Internal Medicine. 2010;**49**:1103-1109

[56] Sugimoto M, Furuta T. Efficacy of tailored *Helicobacter pylori* eradication therapy based on antibiotic

susceptibility and CYP2C19 genotype. World Journal of Gastroenterology. 2014;**20**:6400-6411

[57] Dinis-Ribeiro M, Areia M, de Vries AC, et al. Management of precancerous conditions and lesions in the stomach (MAPS): Guideline from the European Society of Gastrointestinal Endoscopy (ESGE), European Helicobacter Study Group (EHSG), European Society of Pathology (ESP), and the Sociedade Portuguesa. Endoscopy. 2012;**44**:74-94

[58] Leja M, Kupcinskas L, Funka K, et al. Value of gastrin-17 in detecting antral atrophy. Advances in Medical Sciences. 2011;**56**:145-150

[59] McNicholl AG, Forné M, Barrio J, et al. Accuracy of GastroPanel for the diagnosis of atrophic gastritis. European Journal of Gastroenterology & Hepatology. 2014;**26**:941-948

[60] Leodolter A, Domínguez-Muñoz JE, von Arnim U, et al. Validity of a modified 13C-urea breath test for pre- and posttreatment diagnosis of *Helicobacter pylori* infection in the routine clinical setting. The American Journal of Gastroenterology. 1999;**94**:2100-2104

[61] Vaira D, Vakil N, Menegatti M, et al. The stool antigen test for detection of *Helicobacter pylori* after eradication therapy. Annals of Internal Medicine. 2002;**136**:280-287

[62] Chey WD, Metz DC, Shaw S, et al. Appropriate timing of the 14C-urea breath test to establish eradication of *Helicobacter pylori* infection. The American Journal of Gastroenterology. 2000;**95**:1171-1174

[63] Neil GA, Suchower LJ, Ronca PD, et al. Time of *Helicobacter pylori* eradication assessment following treatment. Helicobacter. 1997;**2**:13-20

[64] Chey WD, Leontiadis GI, Howde CW, et al. ACG Clinical Guideline: Treatment of *Helicobacter pylori* infection. The American Journal of Gastroenterology. 2017;**112**:212-238. DOI: 10.1038/ajg.2016.563

[65] Thung I, Aramin H, Vavinskaya V, et al. Review article: The global emergence of *Helicobacter pylori* antibiotic resistance. Alimentary Pharmacology & Therapeutics. 2016;**43**:514-533

[66] Kobayashi I, Murakami K, Kato M, et al. Changing antimicrobial susceptibility epidemiology of *Helicobacter pylori* strains in Japan between 2002 and 2005. Journal of Clinical Microbiology. 2007;**45**:4006-4010

[67] Lee JW, Kim N, Kim JM, et al. Prevalence of primary and secondary antimicrobial resistance of *Helicobacter pylori* in Korea from 2003 through 2012. Helicobacter. 2013;**18**:206-214

[68] Khademi F, Poursina F, Hosseini E, et al. *Helicobacter pylori* in Iran: A systematic review on the antibiotic resistance. Iranian Journal of Basic Medical Sciences. 2015;**18**:2-7

[69] Karamanolis GP, Daikos GL, Xouris D, et al. The evolution of *Helicobacter pylori* antibiotic resistance over 10 years in Greece. Digestion. 2014;**90**:229-231

[70] Megraud F, Coenen S, Versporten A, et al. *Helicobacter pylori* resistance to antibiotics in Europe and its relationship to antibiotic consumption. Gut. 2013;**62**:34-42

[71] Boyanova L, Gergova G, Evstatiev I, et al. *Helicobacter pylori* resistance to six antibiotics by two breakpoint systems and resistance evolution in Bulgaria. Infectious Diseases (London). 2016;**48**:56-62

[72] Nishizawa T, Maekawa T, Watanabe N, et al. Clarithromycin versus metronidazole as first-line *Helicobacter pylori* eradication: A multicenter, prospective, randomized controlled study in Japan. Journal of Clinical Gastroenterology. 2015;**49**:468-471

[73] Graham DY, Lee YC, Wu MS. Rational *Helicobacter pylori* therapy: Evidence-based medicine rather than medicine-based evidence. Clinical Gastroenterology and Hepatology. 2014;**12**:177-186

[74] Molina-Infante J, Gisbert JP. Optimizing clarithromycin-containing therapy for *Helicobacter pylori* in the era of antibiotic resistance. World Journal of Gastroenterology. 2014;**20**:10338-10347

[75] Federico A, Nardone G, Gravina AG, et al. Efficacy of 5-day levofloxacin-containing concomitant therapy in eradication of *Helicobacter pylori* infection. Gastroenterology. 2012;**143**:55.e1-61.e1; quiz e13-14

[76] Toracchio S, Capodicasa S, Soraja DB, et al. Rifabutin based triple therapy for eradication of *H. pylori* primary and secondary resistant to tinidazole and clarithromycin. Digestive and Liver Disease. 2005;**37**:33-38

[77] Ince AT, Tozlu M, Baysal B, et al. Yields of dual therapy containing high-dose proton pump inhibitor in eradication of *H. pylori* positive dyspeptic patients. Hepato-Gastroenterology. 2014;**61**:1454-1458

[78] Liang X, Xu X, Zheng Q, et al. Efficacy of bismuth-containing quadruple therapies for clarithromycin-, metronidazole-, and fluoroquinolone-resistant *Helicobacter pylori* infections in a prospective study. Clinical Gastroenterology and Hepatology. 2013;**11**:802.e1-807. e1

[79] Liu WZ, Xie Y, Cheng H, et al. Fourth Chinese National Consensus Report on the management of *Helicobacter pylori* infection. Journal of Digestive Diseases. 2013;**14**:211-221

[80] Fischbach L, Evans EL. Meta-analysis: The effect of antibiotic resistance status on the efficacy of triple and quadruple first-line therapies for *Helicobacter pylori*. Alimentary Pharmacology & Therapeutics. 2007;**26**:343-357

[81] Graham DY, Shiotani A. Which therapy for *Helicobacter pylori* infection? Gastroenterology. 2012;**143**:10-12

[82] Salazar CO, Cardenas VM, Reddy RK, et al. Greater than 95% success with 14-day bismuth quadruple anti- *Helicobacter pylori* therapy: A pilot study in US Hispanics. Helicobacter. 2012;**17**:382-390

[83] Rimbara E, Fischbach LA, Graham DY. Optimal therapy for *Helicobacter pylori* infections. Nature Reviews. Gastroenterology & Hepatology. 2011;**8**:79-88

[84] Lu H, Zhang W, Graham DY. Bismuth-containing quadruple therapy for *Helicobacter pylori*: Lessons from China. European Journal of Gastroenterology & Hepatology. 2013;**25**:1134-1140

[85] Liou JM, Chen CC, Chen MJ, et al. Sequential versus triple therapy for the first-line treatment of *Helicobacter pylori*: A multicentre, open-label, randomised trial. Lancet. 2013;**381**:205-213

[86] Gatta L, Vakil N, Vaira D, et al. Global eradication rates for *Helicobacter pylori* infection: Systematic review and meta-analysis of sequential therapy. BMJ. 2013;**347**:f4587

[87] Tang HL, Li Y, Hu YF, et al. Effects of CYP2C19 loss-of-function variants

on the eradication of *H. pylori* infection in patients treated with proton pump inhibitor-based triple therapy regimens: A meta-analysis of randomized clinical trials. PLoS One. 2013;**8**:e62162

[88] Padol S, Yuan Y, Thabane M, et al. The effect of CYP2C19 polymorphisms on *H. pylori* eradication rate in dual and triple first-line PPI therapies: A meta-analysis. The American Journal of Gastroenterology. 2006;**101**:1467-1475

[89] Zhao F, Wang J, Yang Y, et al. Effect of CYP2C19 genetic polymorphisms on the efficacy of proton pump inhibitor-based triple therapy for *Helicobacter pylori* eradication: A meta-analysis. Helicobacter. 2008;**13**:532-541

[90] McNicholl AG, Linares PM, Nyssen OP, et al. Meta-analysis: Esomeprazole or rabeprazole vs. first-generation pump inhibitors in the treatment of *Helicobacter pylori* infection. Alimentary Pharmacology & Therapeutics. 2012;**36**:414-425

[91] Tokoro C, Inamori M, Koide T, et al. Does pretreatment with proton pump inhibitors influence the eradication rate of *Helicobacter pylori*? Hepato-Gastroenterology. 2010;**57**:1645-1649

[92] Yoon SB, Park JM, Lee JY, et al. Long-term pretreatment with proton pump inhibitor and *Helicobacter pylori* eradication rates. World Journal of Gastroenterology. 2014;**20**:1061-1066

[93] Labenz J. Current role of acid suppressants in *Helicobacter pylori* eradication therapy. Best Practice & Research. Clinical Gastroenterology. 2001;**15**:413-431

[94] Marin AC, McNicholl AG, Gisbert JP. A review of rescue regimens after clarithromycin-containing triple therapy failure (for *Helicobacter pylori* eradication). Expert Opinion on Pharmacotherapy. 2013;**14**:843-861

[95] Gisbert JP, Morena F. Systematic review and meta-analysis: Levofloxacin-based rescue regimens after *Helicobacter pylori* treatment failure. Alimentary Pharmacology & Therapeutics. 2006;**23**:35-44

[96] Saad RJ, Schoenfeld P, Kim HM, et al. Levofloxacin-based triple therapy versus bismuth-based quadruple therapy for persistent *Helicobacter pylori* infection: A meta-analysis. The American Journal of Gastroenterology. 2006;**101**:488-496

[97] Di Caro S, Fini L, Daoud Y, et al. Levofloxacin/amoxicillin-based schemes vs quadruple therapy for *Helicobacter pylori* eradication in second-line. World Journal of Gastroenterology. 2012;**18**:5669-5678

[98] Saracino IM, Zullo A, Holton J, et al. High prevalence of primary antibiotic resistance in *Helicobacter pylori* isolates in Italy. Journal of Gastrointestinal and Liver Diseases. 2012;**21**:363-365

[99] Gisbert JP, Romano M, Gravina AG, et al. *Helicobacter pylori* second-line rescue therapy with levofloxacin- and bismuth-containing quadruple therapy, after failure of standard triple or non-bismuth quadruple treatments. Alimentary Pharmacology & Therapeutics. 2015;**41**:768-775

[100] Malfertheiner P. Infection: Bismuth improves PPI-based triple therapy for *H. pylori* eradication. Nature Reviews. Gastroenterology & Hepatology. 2010;**7**:538-539

[101] Liao J, Zheng Q, Liang X, et al. Effect of fluoroquinolone resistance on 14-day levofloxacin triple and triple plus bismuth quadruple therapy. Helicobacter. 2013;**18**:373-377

[102] Malfertheiner P, Link A, Selgrad M. *Helicobacter pylori*: Perspectives and time trends. Nature Reviews.

Gastroenterology & Hepatology. 2014;**11**:628-638

[103] López-Góngora S, Puig I, Calvet X, et al. Systematic review and meta-analysis: Susceptibility-guided versus empirical antibiotic treatment for *Helicobacter pylori* infection. The Journal of Antimicrobial Chemotherapy. 2015;**70**:2447-2455

[104] Collen MJ, Johnson DA, Sheridan MJ. Basal acid output and gastric acid hypersecretion in gastroesophageal reflux disease. Correlation with ranitidine therapy. Digestive Diseases and Sciences. 1994;**39**(2):410-417

[105] Gardner JD, Sloan S, Robinson M, Miner PB Jr. Frequency analyses of gastric pH in control and gastro-oesophageal reflux disease subjects treated with a proton-pump inhibitor. Alimentary Pharmacology & Therapeutics. 2004;**20**(11-12):1381-1386. DOI: 10.1111/j.1365-2036.2004.02279.x

[106] Lao-Sirieix P, Corovic A, Jankowski J, Lowe A, Triadafilopoulos G, Fitzgerald RC. Physiological and molecular analysis of acid loading mechanisms in squamous and *Helicobacter pylori* and extragastric diseases 343 columnar-lined esophagus. Diseases of the Esophagus. 2008;**21**(6):529-538. DOI: 10.1111/j.1442-2050.2007.00807.x

[107] Runge TM, Abrams JA, Shaheen NJ. Epidemiology of Barrett's esophagus and esophageal adenocarcinoma. Gastroenterology Clinics of North America. 2015;**44**(2):203-231. DOI: 10.1016/j.gtc.2015.02.001

[108] Rubenstein JH, Inadomi JM, Scheiman J, Schoenfeld P, Appelman H, Zhang M, et al. Association between *Helicobacter pylori* and Barrett's esophagus, erosive esophagitis, *Helicobacter pylori* and extragastric diseases 345 and gastroesophageal reflux symptoms. Clinical Gastroenterology and Hepatology. 2014;**12**(2):239-245. DOI: 10.1016/j.cgh.2013.08.029

[109] Chung H, Pamp SJ, Hill JA, Surana NK, Edelman SM, Troy EB, et al. Gut immune maturation depends on colonization with a host-specific microbiota. Cell. 2012;**149**:1578-1593. DOI: 10.1016/j.cell.2012.04.037

[110] Minatsuki C, Yamamichi N, Shimamoto T, Kakimoto H, Takahashi Y, Fujishiro M, et al. Background factors of reflux esophagitis and non-erosive reflux disease: A cross-sectional study of 10,837 subjects in Japan. PLoS One. 2013;**8**(7):e69891. DOI: 10.1371/journal.pone.0069891

[111] Fischbach LA, Nordenstedt H, Kramer JR, Gandhi S, Dick-Onuoha S, Lewis A, et al. The association between Barrett's esophagus and *Helicobacter pylori* infection: A meta-analysis. Helicobacter. 2012;**17**(3):163-175. DOI: 10.1111/j.1523-5378.2011.00931.x

[112] Nie S, Chen T, Yang X, Huai P, Lu M. Association of *Helicobacter pylori* infection with esophageal adenocarcinoma and squamous cell carcinoma: A meta-analysis. Diseases of the Esophagus. 2014;**27**(7):645-653. DOI: 10.1111/dote.12194

[113] Baumgart DC, Bernstein CN, Abbas Z, Colombel JF, Day AS, D'Haens G, et al. IBD around the world: Comparing the epidemiology, diagnosis, and treatment: Proceedings of the World Digestive Health Day 2010—Inflammatory bowel disease task force meeting. Inflammatory Bowel Diseases. 2011;**17**(2):639-644. DOI: 10.1002/ibd.21409

[114] Pearce CB, Duncan HD, Timmis L, Green JR. Assessment of the prevalence of infection with *Helicobacter pylori*

in patients with inflammatory bowel disease. European Journal of Gastroenterology & Hepatology. 2000;**12**(4):439-443

[115] Pronai L, Schandl L, Orosz Z, Magyar P, Tulassay Z. Lower prevalence of *Helicobacter pylori* infection in patients with inflammatory bowel disease but not with chronic obstructive pulmonary disease—Antibiotic use in the history does not play a significant role. Helicobacter. 2004;**9**(3):278-283. DOI: 10.1111/j.1083-4389.2004.00223.xHEL223

[116] Piodi LP, Bardella M, Rocchia C, Cesana BM, Baldassarri A, Quatrini M. Possible protective effect of 5-aminosalicylic acid on *Helicobacter pylori* infection in patients with inflammatory bowel disease. Journal of Clinical Gastroenterology. 2003;**36**(1):22-25

[117] Wu XW, Ji HZ, Yang MF, Wu L, Wang FY. *Helicobacter pylori* infection and inflammatory bowel disease in Asians: A meta-analysis. World Journal of Gastroenterology. 2015;**21**(15): 4750-4756. DOI: 10.3748/wjg.v21.i15.4750

[118] Rokkas T, Gisbert JP, Niv Y, O'Morain C. The association between *Helicobacter pylori* infection and inflammatory bowel disease based on meta-analysis. United European Gastroenterology Journal. 2015;**3**(6):539-550. DOI: 10.1177/2050 64061558088910.1177_205064061558 0889

[119] Castano-Rodriguez N, Kaakoush NO, Lee WS, Mitchell HM. Dual role of *Helicobacter* and *Campylobacter* species in IBD: A systematic review and meta-analysis. Gut. Feb 2017;**66**(2):235-249. DOI: 10.1136/gutjnl-2015-310545

[120] Andersson AF, Lindberg M, Jakobsson H, et al. Comparative analysis of human gut microbiota by barcoded pyrosequencing. PLoS One. 2008;**3**:e2836

[121] Bik EM, Eckburg PB, Gill SR, et al. Molecular analysis of the bacterial microbiota in the human stomach. Proceedings of the National Academy of Sciences of the United States of America. 2006;**103**:732-737

[122] Li XX, Wong GLH, To KF, et al. Bacterial microbiota profiling in gastritis without *Helicobacter pylori* infection or non-steroidal anti-inflammatory drug use. PLoS One. 2009;**4**:e7985

[123] Yang I, Nell S, Suerbaum S. Survival in hostile territory: The microbiota of the stomach. FEMS Microbiology Reviews. 2013;**37**:736-761

[124] Yang I, Woltemate S, Piazuelo MB, et al. Different gastric microbiota compositions in two human populations with high and low gastric cancer risk in Colombia. Scientific Reports. 2016;**6**:18594

[125] Debongnie JC, Donnay M, Mairesse J, et al. Gastric ulcers and *Helicobacter heilmannii*. European Journal of Gastroenterology & Hepatology. 1998;**10**:251-254

[126] Matsumoto T, Kawakubo M, Akamatsu T, et al. Helicobacter heilmannii sensu stricto-related gastric ulcers: A case report. World Journal of Gastroenterology. 2014;**20**:3376-3382

[127] Morgner A, Bayerdörffer E, Meining A, et al. *Helicobacter heilmannii* and gastric cancer. Lancet. 1995;**346**:511-512

[128] Morgner A, Lehn N, Andersen LP, et al. *Helicobacter heilmannii*-associated primary gastric low-grade MALT lymphoma: Complete remission after

curing the infection. Gastroenterology. 2000;**118**:821-828

[129] Haesebrouck F, Pasmans F, Flahou B, et al. Gastric Helicobacters in domestic animals and nonhuman primates and their significance for human health. Clinical Microbiology Reviews. 2009;**22**:202-223

[130] Stolte M, Kroher G, Meining A, et al. A comparison of *Helicobacter pylori* and *H. heilmannii* gastritis. A matched control study involving 404 patients. Scandinavian Journal of Gastroenterology. 1997;**32**:28-33

[131] Ladirat SE, Schols HA, Nauta A, et al. High-throughput analysis of the impact of antibiotics on the human intestinal microbiota composition. Journal of Microbiological Methods. 2013;**92**:387-397

[132] Marteau P, Rambaud JC. Potential of using lactic acid bacteria for therapy and immunomodulation in man. FEMS Microbiology Reviews. 1993;**12**:207-220

[133] Lessa FC, Mu Y, Bamberg WM, et al. Burden of *Clostridium difficile* infection in the United States. The New England Journal of Medicine. 2015;**372**:825-834

[134] Dang Y, Reinhardt JD, Zhou X, et al. The effect of probiotics supplementation on *Helicobacter pylori* eradication rates and side effects during eradication therapy: A meta-analysis. PLoS One. 2014;**9**:e111030

[135] Lv Z, Wang B, Zhou X, et al. Efficacy and safety of probiotics as adjuvant agents for *Helicobacter pylori* infection: A meta-analysis. Experimental and Therapeutic Medicine. 2015;**9**:707-716

[136] Tong JL, Ran ZH, Shen J, et al. Meta-analysis: The effect of supplementation with probiotics on eradication rates and adverse events during *Helicobacter pylori* eradication therapy. Alimentary Pharmacology & Therapeutics. 2007;**25**:155-168

[137] Wang ZH, Gao QY, Fang JY. Meta-analysis of the efficacy and safety of Lactobacillus-containing and Bifidobacterium-containing probiotic compound preparation in *Helicobacter pylori* eradication therapy. Journal of Clinical Gastroenterology. 2013;**47**:25-32

[138] Zhang M-M, Qian W, Qin Y-Y, et al. Probiotics in *Helicobacter pylori* eradication therapy: A systematic review and meta-analysis. World Journal of Gastroenterology. 2015;**21**:4345-4357

[139] Zheng X, Lyu L, Mei Z. Lactobacillus-containing probiotic supplementation increases *Helicobacter pylori* eradication rate: Evidence from a meta-analysis. Revista Española de Enfermedades Digestivas. 2013;**105**:445-453

[140] Zhu R, Chen K, Zheng Y-Y, et al. Meta-analysis of the efficacy of probiotics in *Helicobacter pylori* eradication therapy. World Journal of Gastroenterology. 2014;**20**:18013-18021

[141] Zou J, Dong J, Yu X. Meta-analysis: Lactobacillus containing quadruple therapy versus standard triple first-line therapy for *Helicobacter pylori* eradication. Helicobacter. 2009;**14**:97-107

[142] Vladimirov B. Treatment of helicobacter-pylori associated diseases. In: Boyanova L, editor. Helicobacter pylori. Norfolk, UK: Caister Academic Press; 2011:237-251

[143] Li S, Huang XL, Sui JZ, et al. Meta-analysis of randomized controlled trials on the efficacy of probiotics in *Helicobacter pylori* eradication therapy in children. European Journal of Pediatrics. 2014;**173**:153-161

[144] Sachdeva A, Nagpal J. Effect of fermented milk-based probiotic preparations on *Helicobacter pylori* eradication: A systematic review and meta-analysis of randomized-controlled trials. European Journal of Gastroenterology & Hepatology. 2009;**21**:45-53

[145] Szajewska H, Horvath A, Kołodziej M. Systematic review with meta-analysis: *Saccharomyces boulardii* supplementation and eradication of *Helicobacter pylori* infection. Alimentary Pharmacology & Therapeutics. 2015;**41**:1237-1245

Chapter 2

Helicobacter pylori: A Pathogen of Ample Risk to Health

Isidro Favian Bayas-Morejón, Rosa Angélica Tigre-León, Edison Riveliño Ramón-Curay and Darwin Alberto Núñez-Torres

Abstract

Helicobacter pylori is considered a pathogen of global interest because it is a microorganism of very easy contagion between the hosts or host. *Helicobacter pylori* infection is now recognized as a problem that causes chronic gastritis, peptic ulcer disease, and lymphoproliferative disorders and is a major risk factor for gastric cancer. The diagnostic methods to detect *H. pylori* are classified such as direct or invasive, when the identification is directly, the bacterium obtained from gastric mucosa biopsy by endoscopy histology with various staining, culture and PCR techniques, while indirect or noninvasive or serological tests such as the breath test with urea marked with 13C.

Keywords: *H. pylori*, pathogen, risk to human

1. Introduction

Helicobacter pylori is considered a pathogen of global interest because it is a microorganism of very easy contagion between hosts or susceptible hosts. The first isolation of *H. pylori* was in 1982 by Marshall and Warren who ushered us into a new era of gastric microbiology [1].

The number of infected by *H. pylori* has been increased considerably, since a third of the world population has it, while the rest do not know if they have it or not; in developing countries there is an infection rate that goes from 60% and 90% of the population, which is not the case in developed countries ranging from 20–40% [2]. Gastroduodenal ulcer diseases are a major factor in the development of gastric adenocarcinoma and lymphoma [3].

According to studies conducted, many of the pathogenic species of *Helicobacter* are of fecal origin. The transmission to human seems to be associated with the consumption of water and raw or undercooked foods [4, 5]. In Ecuador, according to the statistics, the poverty quintiles reached up to 2015 are 35% according to INEC data, which are closely related to the lack of basic services such as drinking water and sanitary services, a common factor in the population being contamination by water and food [6].

The different methods used for diagnosis range from antigenic screening (Ag) to molecular techniques. Antigenic screening techniques have been associated with a high sensitivity of a detection limit of the *Helicobacter pylori* test with a 95% concordance in specificity compared to the ELISA test [7]. In plate culture it is usually considered a difficult and tedious technique; the diagnostic method has the advantage of typifying the organism and determining its sensitivity to antibacterial agents. The methods such as endoscopy to obtain a sample through a biopsy are very used nowadays; it is a traumatic and invasive procedure that can cause complications such as infections, perforations, aspiration, bleeding, and incarceration of the endoscope [8].

2. Theoretical framework

2.1 *Helicobacter pylori*

Helicobacter pylori (*H. pylori*) is a spiral bacterium that does not form spores and is Gram-negative, which colonizes the human stomach and is prevalent throughout the world [9]. It has been associated with peptic ulcer disease, gastric adenocarcinoma, and lower grade B-associated lymphoma associated with the mucosa. In addition, it is thought that the organism is involved in other human diseases such as hematological and autoimmune disorders, insulin resistance, and metabolic syndrome [10]. Although almost 50% of the population is infected with *H. pylori* worldwide, the prevalence, incidence, age distribution, and sequelae of infection are significantly different in developed and developing countries.

Helicobacter pylori (previously known as *Campylobacter pylori* or pyloridis) was first isolated from humans in 1982 [11]. Since 1994, *H. pylori* has been considered carcinogenic to humans, and it has even been associated with other diseases, such as cerebrovascular accidents, autoimmune thyroiditis, and diabetes mellitus, among others [12]. This bacterium resides in the stomach of most humans and is usually found in the deeper portions of the mucus gel that lines the gastric mucosa or between the mucus layer and the gastric epithelium [13].

The bacterium is one of the most important findings for gastroenterologists, who for years sought answers to multiple intestinal problems. This is how the gastroenterologist Walery Jaworski in 1899 after analyzing samples of human gastric expirations isolated spiral elongated bacteria and called them *Vibrio regula*, and the said results were published in the manual of gastric diseases; however, these findings were not given the importance they deserved to be written in Polish and not in English [14].

So, it took 79 years for the bacteria to be rediscovered by the Australian doctors Barry Marshall and Robin Warren, who managed to make the first isolation through a pure culture in 1979. This rediscovery allowed them to be Nobel Laureates in 2005 [15].

2.2 Microbiological aspects of *Helicobacter pylori*

Taxonomically, we can describe *H. pylori* because of its size, shape, color, biochemical function, genus, species, and its relationship with other species. *H. pylori* is a slow-growing, spiral-shaped bacterium. It is a small curved bacillus, microaerophilic, and Gram-negative, and mobile by the presence of flagella. The bacillus has rounded ends. These microorganisms measure 0.5–1.0 μm wide by 2.5–4.0 μm long, since they bear a strong resemblance to members of the *Campylobacter* genus [11].

The multiple genotypic and phenotypic characteristics are different from those of *Helicobacter*, so this new genus was established, including *H. cinaedi* and *H. fennelliae*. The two species of *Helicobacter* that cause diarrheal disease, *H. cinaedi* and *H. fennelliae*, are intestinal microorganisms rather than gastric. As for the clinical manifestations of the disease they generate, these bacteria are more similar to *Campylobacter* than *H. pylori* [13]. The clinical characteristics of the infections caused by these *Helicobacter* are similar to those due to *Campylobacter* species.

2.3 Pathways of contagion or infestation of the guests

Although in general there is no difference between the sexes, in some developed countries, there is a higher prevalence of infection in men than in women [16].

The prevalence of *H. pylori* infection in adults of any age in developed countries ranges between 20 and 40% and reaches figures of 60 to 80% in countries considered third world. The most important difference between countries of high and low prevalence is the intensity with which the infection is transmitted in childhood and early adolescence [17].

Epidemiological and microbiological evidences have several transmission routes that have been proposed in the studies carried out. The gastro-oral, oral-oral, and fecal-oral routes are the most important routes of transmission [12]. Other routes of importance are also breastfeeding and iatrogenic transmission which are also included as alternating forms for the transmission of the pathogen. The possibilities of spreading the pathogen are of three possible vectors that have been suggested to maintain the viable form of the bacteria: water, food, and animals.

2.4 Water transmission

The prevalence of *H. pylori* infection shows a strong correlation with access to water. Numerous epidemiological studies confirm this, and the World Health Organization includes it in its list of potential emerging pathogenic microorganisms whose transmission by water is plausible, although it has not yet been confirmed [18, 19].

Through molecular methods, *H. pylori* DNA has been detected in wastewater, drinking water, and other environmental samples throughout the world, and its survival capacity in water, even chlorinated, has been demonstrated. It has also been detected in the drinking water distribution network [20]. These findings indicate that contaminated water and food play a vital role in the survival and spread of *H. pylori*.

In another study, developed by Moreno et al. [21]; Moreno and Ferrús, [22] *H. pylori* was detected in 46% of more than 100 wastewater samples, 40% were of river water samples and, most strikingly, the 66% were public source.

On the other hand, *H. pylori* is able to survive in biofilms when it grows under high C:N conditions [23]. The biofilms formed protect microorganisms from the action of adverse agents, increase the availability of nutrients for their growth, and also increase the frequency of transfer of genetic material [24]. Gião et al. [25] observed that *H. pylori* formed biofilms after 24 hours of being in an unfavorable environment. The association of *H. pylori* with biofilm communities within a water distribution system could offer the bacterium protection against disinfection and predation by protozoa, and there are studies that demonstrate the survival of *H. pylori* within amoebae of free life[26, 27].

2.5 Foods transmission

Those foods that have a water activity (aw) >0.97 and a pH between 4.9 and 6.0 theoretically provide the ideal conditions for the survival and development of *H. pylori* [28, 29].

Vegetables are one of the foods with the highest risk of fecal contamination, since they are in contact with soil and contaminated irrigation water, which would mean the spread of *H. pylori* in the environment and its transmission to humans. Atapoor et al. [30] and Yahaghi et al. [31] in Iran managed to detect and isolate *H. pylori* in percentages higher than 10%, in vegetable samples. Also, Bayas et al. [32] have detected the pathogen in vegetables by molecular methods.

On the other hand, the ability of *H. pylori* to survive on lettuce leaves forming biofilms has been demonstrated [33].

Milk could also act as a vehicle for *H. pylori*. Several studies have shown that the bacterium is able to survive in inoculated milk stored in refrigeration for more than 6 days or for 3 days at room temperature [34]. In addition, in an investigation developed by Fujimura et al. [35], the presence of the *H. pylori* ureA gene was detected in 13 of 18 samples of raw milk (72.2%) and in 11 of 20 samples of pasteurized milk (55%).

On the other hand, Meng et al. [36] analyzed 11 raw chickens and 18 samples of tuna meat ready for consumption (sushi). *H. pylori* was detected by multiple polymerase chain reaction (m-PCR) in 36% (4/11) of the chickens and 44% (8/18) of the tuna samples.

Studies have also been conducted on the presence of *H. pylori* in shellfish. Fernández et al. [37] detected *H. pylori* DNA in seawater, plankton, and oysters from three different regions of Venezuela. They concluded that mollusks could act as vehicles for *H. pylori* transmission.

2.6 Detection in human samples

The presence of *H. Pylori* was focused on a study developed by Samie [38], on the prevalence of *Campylobacter*, *Helicobacter*, and *Arcobacter*. By molecular methods, in 322 stool samples from HIV-positive and non-HIV-infected patients in South Africa, they found that *A. butzleri* was the third most frequent species (6.2%), after *Helicobacter pylori* (50.6%) and *Campylobacter jejuni* (10.2%).

2.7 Most common pathologies

2.7.1 Gastritis

The term gastritis should be reserved for the histologically demonstrated inflammation of the gastric mucosa. Gastritis is not the mucosal erythema seen during endoscopy, nor is it interchangeable with the term "dyspepsia" [13]. On the other hand, the different etiological factors that cause gastritis are multiple and heterogeneous; to gastritis it has been classified with a chronological base (acute or chronic), such as histological typologies, anatomical distribution or its pathogenic mechanism, clinical correlation, histological data, abdominal pain or dyspepsia, and endoscopic data in gastric mucosal investigation [13].

The pathogenesis of chronic gastritis by *Helicobacter pylori* includes two stages: the first is characterized by the arrival and penetration of the microorganism into the gastric mucus where it sits and multiplies. In the second stage, there is an amplification of the inflammatory response, by the interaction of lymphocytes, neutrophils, macrophages, mastoid cells, and nonimmune cells that, when attracted to the site of the lesion, release a wide variety of chemical mediators such as cytokines, eicosanoids, reactive oxygen metabolites (oxygen free radicals), and the complement system, which perpetuate inflammation [39, 40] (**Figure 1**).

2.7.2 Stomach cancer

It is the uncontrolled growth of stomach cells. Malignant tumors can originate in each of the three layers: mucosa, muscle, and serosa. This is also known as gastric cancer that originates in the stomach [41]. The risk factor is considered any caused that increases the likelihood of having a disease such as cancer, even though several risk components do not mean that the person will have the disease; Some scientists connoted that the risks that take a person to be more prone to suffer stomach cancer are several such as:

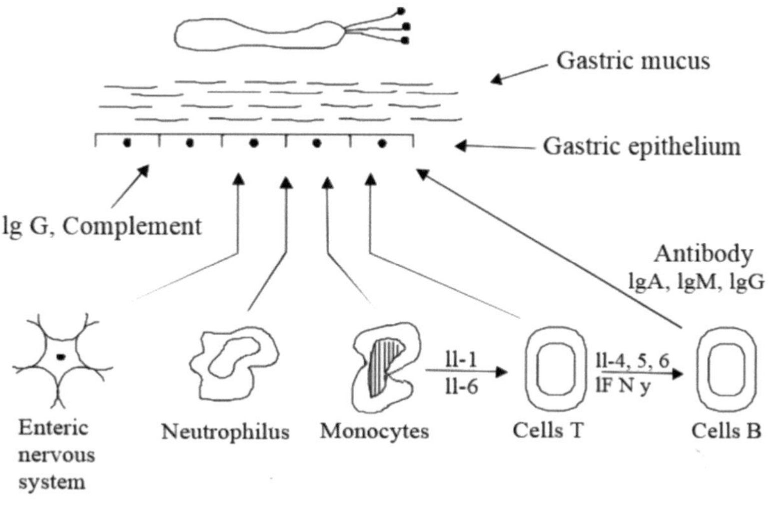

Figure 1.
Second stage of the inflammatory process of the gastric mucosa by H. pylori. Grávalos and González [40].

Incidence according to sex: Stomach cancer is more common in men than in women [16].

Age: The rate of stomach cancer in people over 50 years increases sharply [42].

Ethnic origin: In the United States, stomach cancer is more common among Americans of Hispanic origin, black people, and Asians and islanders compared to white people who are not of Hispanic origin [41].

Geography: On a global scale, stomach cancer is more common in Japan, China, Eastern and Southern Europe, as well as Central and South America [41].

2.7.3 Risk factors

Several risk factors for gastric cancer have been described, which play a fundamental role in their genesis, some of them remain under discussion, and others, on the contrary, have been confirmed more and more clearly [43].

2.7.4 Genetic

Within the genetic risk factors [41], we have:

- Families of patients with gastric cancer: incidence 2–3 times higher
- Blood group A.

2.7.5 Environmental

Among the environmental risk factors [41], we have:

- Food (variable in each country): dried and salted fish, very spicy foods, and red meats, among others
- Ingestion of alcohol, hot drinks, and sodium nitrate; chewed tobacco
- Radiation.

2.7.6 Premalignant

Within the premalignant risk factors [41], we have:

- Atrophic gastritis, intestinal metaplasm, and dysplasia.
- Pernicious anemia (20 times more frequent than in normal subjects).
- Gastric polyps: multiple hyperplasia, greater than 2 cm with some degree of dysplasia 0.4–4% of association with gastric cancer [41].

2.7.7 Stomach lymphoma

People who have suffered from a certain type of stomach lymphoma, known as lymphoma of lymphatic tissue associated with the mucosa (MALT), have an increased risk of developing adenocarcinoma of the stomach, probably due to infection with *H. pylori* [41] (**Figure 2**).

2.7.8 H. pylori and peptic disorders

The gastric infection produced by *H. pylori* bacteria in most cases of peptic ulcer is also important in the appearance of lymphomas that originate in the lymphoid tissue (MALT) and in gastric adenocarcinoma [13]. The peptic ulcer is an ulcer that affects the lining of the stomach and is the causes of internal bleeding of the upper digestive tract with severe complications that lead to an adenocarcinoma [13, 40].

2.7.9 Diagnostic methods of H. pylori infection

The diagnostic methods of *H. pylori* infection have traditionally been classified as direct and indirect; the former is based on the "direct" demonstration of the microorganism by means of the study of samples obtained by gastric biopsy [44]. This technique used is very stressful and uncomfortable for the patient because of the invasive reason.

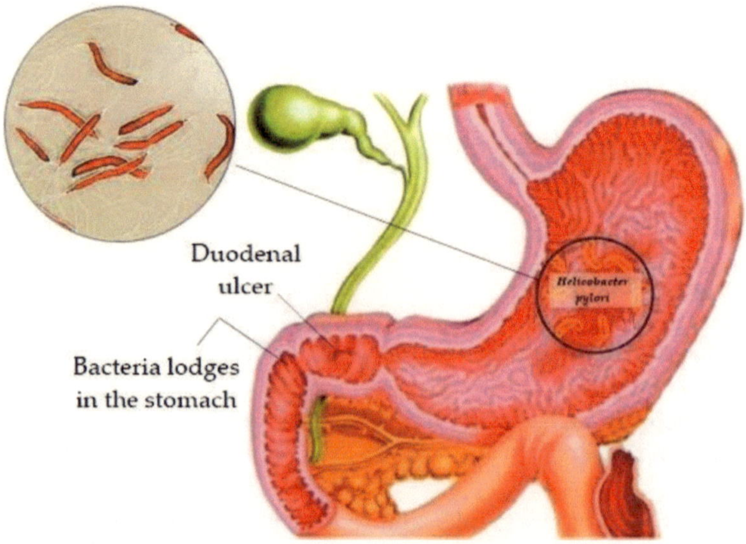

Figure 2.
Entrance and lodging of H. pylori in the stomach. Grávalos and González [40].

The other indirect methods are based on the detection of certain characteristics of the bacteria, such as the ability to hydrolyze through urea, and based on the breath test or the response of the immune system through the measurement of specific antibodies. Its primary advantage is its noninvasive nature [44].

2.7.10 Histological techniques

The presence of the germ can be recognized with the usual hematoxylin and eosin stain, although it is more easily demonstrated with other stains such as Giemsa. The histology not only demonstrates the presence of the microorganism but also informs about the morphological changes of the gastric mucosa [44].

2.7.11 Cultivation of H. pylori

Under optimal conditions *H. pylori* is extremely difficult to grow, due to its demanding nutritional requirements and its slow growth. The cultivation of *H. pylori* is usually slow, the first colonies usually appear between the fifth and seventh days, and it may take up to 10 days. Being a microaerophilic microorganism requires atmospheres with 5–10% of O_2, 5–10% of CO_2, and 80–90% of N_2 at 35–37°C, with a humidity of 90–95% [45].

The selection and inoculation of the bacteria depend on the number and types of tests to be carried out as well as on the factors, type of bacteria, clinical importance of the isolation, availability of the strain, and reliable method of verification [46]. Plate culture has advantages ranging from typifying the organism to determining its sensitivity to antibacterial agents, so it is important to study it from the epidemiological point of view, because it allows knowing the pattern of resistance to different therapeutic regimens with a specificity of the 100% and a lower sensitivity than other diagnostic techniques [3]. This microorganism is also urease, oxidase, and catalase positive, characteristics that are frequently used in the identification of the microorganism, although its isolation is relatively complex [16].

It is usually considered a difficult and tedious technique. However, adopting a series of minimal precautions, most laboratories achieve the growth of the microorganism [44].

2.7.12 Serology

Serological techniques only indicate a previous exposure to the microorganism but do not discriminate between people with active infection and disease in healthy individuals with prior exposure to infection [44]. Rapid tests are methods for the detection of antigens and antibodies in serum, plasma, whole blood, and other fluids, which give results in a few minutes [47]. These serological techniques are widely used today for rapid diagnosis in laboratories.

The enzyme-linked immunosorbent assay (ELISA) is widely used to perform epidemiological studies on a considerable number of individuals [48].

In a work done by Siavoshi et al. [49], for the intracellular detection of *H. pylori* in yeast identified in oral samples of newborns, the authors detected *H. pylori* with immunofluorescence using polyclonal antibodies IgG anti-*H. pylori* in a rabbit labeled with FITC, whose concentration was 5000 mg/ml, with a wavelength of 528 nm.

2.7.13 Antigenic screening

This is a chromatographic immunoassay for the qualitative detection of *H. pylori* antigen in human stool samples, with a relative sensitivity of 94%, a specificity of 95%, and an accuracy of 97.5%, since it is an in vitro technique ad-bio [50].

Methods	Characteristic	Advantage	Disadvantages
Direct			
Histological techniques	Habitual staining of hematoxylin and eosin Giemsa stain	Demonstrates the presence of the microorganism and reports on changes in the mucosa	The technique requires samples obtained from a biopsy Proper selection of stain fixatives
Direct and indirect			
Culture	Cultivation of the microorganism in specific media under microaerobic conditions The optimum temperature of culture is from 35 to 37°C [53]	Isolate the microorganism to study its behavior (in vitro)	It is difficult to isolate, since *H. pylori* is very sensitive to drying and to the usual atmospheric conditions (it requires the transport of samples in the shortest possible time) [54]. Samples destined for culture remain viable for approximately 5 hours and when stored in saline at 4°C or for more than 24 hours if stored at 4°C in a transport medium specific for *H. pylori* [55] Another disadvantage is the high contamination of the environment with accompanying biota, which makes it difficult to isolate *H. pylori* independently
Indirect			
Serological techniques	Methods for the detection of antigens and antibodies (serum, plasma, and whole blood, among others) Enzyme-linked immunosorbent assay (ELISA)	Rapid laboratory tests	It can induce a false-negative result
Antigenic screening	Chromatographic immunoassay for the detection of *H. pylori* antigens in stool samples	Rapid laboratory tests	Possible false positives due to cross reactions with other organisms [56]
Molecular Methods	DNA amplification of the pathogen	Great versatility as an analysis technique, sequences are amplified from minute amounts of target DNA, even from DNA contained in a single cell	Need to have information on the target DNA sequence Short size of the PCR products The ease with which DNA is amplified requires avoiding the danger of contamination inherent to the multiplier power of the reaction

Table 1.
Comparison of diagnostic methods for H. pylori.

2.7.14 Molecular methods

Molecular methods are the names given to all the laboratory techniques used to isolate DNA or extract it in high purity, visualize it to see its state, cut it and paste it (Iglesias [51]), or amplify a region in a huge amount of molecules: fragment cloning in bacteria or other vectors such as viruses as well as polymerase chain reaction (PCR).

Infectious diseases have become the "spearhead" for the development of molecular diagnostic tests, with more than 50% of the techniques available today. The main explanation for this development is due to the difficulty of detecting a pathogen through classical microbiology [52] (**Table 1**).

3. Conclusion

H. pylori is a microorganism of global interest, given that, in developing countries, the infection overcomes the 60%. Besides, being microorganisms of difficult isolation, the used techniques to culture are insufficient, so that molecular methods and antigen screening are the most recommended for detection, since these techniques are not invasive to patients.

Author details

Isidro Favian Bayas-Morejón*, Rosa Angélica Tigre-León,
Edison Riveliño Ramón-Curay and Darwin Alberto Núñez-Torres
Universidad Estatal de Bolívar, Facultad de Ciencias Agropecuarias Recursos Naturales y del Ambiente, Centro de Investigación y Desarrollo Biotecnológico

*Address all correspondence to: favian_bm@hotmail.com

References

[1] Cava F, Cobas FC. Dos décadas de *Helicobacter pylori*. Scielo. 2003;**12**(1):1-10

[2] Rodríguez Br, González JJ, Carpio L. Tratamiento para Erradicación de en una población salvadoreña Terapia Secuencial vs Triple Terapia Convencional [tesis doctoral]. 2012

[3] Gisbert J, Molina-Infante J. Tratamiento actual de la infección por *Helicobacter pylori*. Medicina Clínica (Barcelona). 2017;**148**:20-22

[4] Bayas Morejón F. Aportaciones a la epidemiología de arcobacter y helicobaaplicación de métodos moleculares a su detección e identificación en alimentos [Tesis Doctoral]. Valencia: Politecnica de Valencia. 2016

[5] Guamán JF, Bayas-Morejón F, Arcos V, Tigre-León A, Lucio-Quintana A, Salazar S, et al. Detection of *Helicobacter pylori* from human biological samples (Feces) by antigenic screening and culture. Jundishapur Journal of Microbiology. 2018;**11**(7):e66721

[6] Dirección Nacional de Vigilancia Epidemiológica_MSP—Ecuador. *Anuario*. Obtenido de Enfermedades Trasmitidas Por Agua Y Alimentos. 2017. https://public.tableau.com/profile/vvicentee80#!/vizhome/ETAS-2014/ANUARIO

[7] Linear Chemicals S.L. 2017. Website. Obtenido de: http://www.linear.es/ficheros/archivos/481_4245125H.PyloriAgcassette25tcas.pdf

[8] Fundacion Española de Endoscopia Digestiva. 2009. Complicaciones de la Endoscopia Digestiva Alta. Protocolos y Directrices en Endoscopia

[9] Smolka AJ, Backert SJ. How *Helicobacter pylori* infection controls gastric acid secretion. Gastroenterology. 2012;**47**(6):609-618

[10] Hasni SA. Role of *Helicobacter pylori* infection in autoimmune diseases. Current Opinion in Rheumatology. 2012;**24**(4):429-434

[11] Mandell R. Enfermedades infecciosas Principios y Practicas. España: Elsevier España, S.L; 2012

[12] Palomino E. Manuales Venezolanos de Nutrición. Obtenido de Helicobacter pylori: Rol del agua y los alimentos en su transmisión. 2016. http://www.scielo.org.ve/scielo.php?script=sci_arttext&pid=S0798075220120002000O5

[13] Harrison. Medicina interna volumen 2. España: Mcgraw-hill interamericana editores, s. A. de C. V. 2012. p. 125

[14] Konturek JW. Discovery by Jaworski of *Helicobacter pylori* and its pathogenetic role inpeptic ulcer, gastritis and cancer gastric. Journal of Physiology and Pharmacology. 2003;**54**(3):23-41

[15] Novo Villaverde FJ. GENÉTICA HUMANA Conceptos, Mecanismos y Aplicaciones de la Genética en el campo de la Biomedicina (Vol. 1ra EDICION). pearson prentice hall. 2007. ISBN: 978-848-322-359-8

[16] Martel C, Parsonnet J. *Helicobacter pylori* infection and gender: A meta-analysis of population-based prevalence surveys. Digestive Diseases and Sciences. 2006;**51**(12):2292-2230

[17] Figueroa G, Troncoso M, Toledo MS, Faúndez G, Acuña R. Prevalence of serum antibodies to *Helicobacter pylori* VacA and CagA and gastric diseases in Chile. Journal of Medical Microbiology. 2002;**51**(4):300-304

[18] Aziz RK, Khalifa MM, Sharaf RR. Contaminated water as a source of *Helicobacter pylori* infection: A review. Journal of Advanced Research. 2015;**6**(4):539-547

[19] Santiago P, Moreno Y, Ferrús MA. Identification of viable *helicobacter pylori* in drinking water supplies by cultural and molecular techniques. Helicobacter. 2015;**20**(4):252-259

[20] Eusebi LH, Zagari RM, Bazzoli F. Epidemiology of *Helicobacter pylori* infection. Helicobacter. 2014;**19** (Suppl 1):1-5

[21] Moreno Y, Ferrús MA, Alonso JL, Jiménez A, y Hernández J. Use of fluorescent in situ hybridization to evidence the presence of *Helicobacter pylori* in water. Water Research, 2003;**37**(9):2251-2256

[22] Moreno Y, Ferrus MA. Specific detection of cultivable *Helicobacter pylori* cells from wastewater treatment plants. Helicobacter. 2012;**17**(5):327-332

[23] Percival SL, Suleman L. Biofilms and *Helicobacter pylori*: Dissemination and persistence within the environment and host. World Journal of Gastrointestinal Pathophysiology. 2014;**5**(3):122-132

[24] Donlan RM. Biofilms: Microbial life on surfaces. Emerging Infectious Diseases. 2002;**8**(9):881-890

[25] Gião MS, Azevedo NF, Wilks SA, Vieira MJ, Keevil CW. Persistence of *Helicobacter pylori* in heterotrophic drinking-water biofilms. Applied and Environmental Microbiology. 2008;**74**(19):5898-5904

[26] Watson CL, Owen RJ, Said B, Lai S, Lee JV, Surman-Lee S, et al. Detection of *Helicobacter pylori* by PCR but not culture in water and biofilm samples from drinking water distribution systems in England. Journal of Applied Microbiology. 2004;**97**(4):690-698

[27] Moreno-Mesonero L, Moreno Y, Alonso JL, Ferrús MA. DVC-FISH and PMA-qPCR techniques to assess the survival of *Helicobacter pylori* inside *Acanthamoeba castellanii*. Research in Microbiology. 2016;**167**(1):29-34

[28] Van-Duynhoven YTHP, De-Jonge R. Transmission of *Helicobacter pylori*: A role for food. Bulletin of the World Health Organization. 2001;**79**(5):455-460

[29] Beuchat LR. Ecological factors influencing survival and growth of human pathogens on raw fruits and vegetables. Microbes and Infection. 2002;**4**(4):413-423

[30] Atapoor S, Safarpoor Dehkordi F, Rahimi E. Detection of *Helicobacter pylori* in various types of vegetables and salads. Jundishapur Journal of Microbiology. 2014;7(5):e10013

[31] Yahaghi E, Khamesipour F, Mashayekhi F, Safarpoor Dehkordi F, Hossein SM, Masoudimanesh M, et al. *Helicobacter pylori* in vegetables and salads: Genotyping and antimicrobial resistance properties. BioMed Research International. 2014;**1**:11. Article ID: 757941

[32] Bayas-Morejón IF, González A, Moreno-Mesonero L, Moreno Y, Ferrús M. Detection of *Helicobacter pylori* in vegetables, XXIXth international workshop on *Helicobacter* and microbiota in inflammation on & cancer, Magdeburg-Germany. Helicobacter. 2016;**21**(Suppl 1):69-177. DOI: 10.1111/hel.12344. [PubMed: 27531543]

[33] Ng CG, Hassanbhai AM, Loke MF, Wong HJ, Goh KL, Vadivelu J, et al. *Helicobacter pylori* biofilm—The probable mode and source of transmission? Helicobacter. 2014;**19**(Suppl 1):104

[34] Boehmler G, Gerwert J, Scupin E, Sinell HJ. Epidemiology of *H. pylori* in man: Studies on the survival of the agent in food. Deutsche Medizinische Wochenschrift. 1996;**103**:438-443

[35] Fujimura S, Kawamura T, Kato S, Tateno H, Wanatabe A. Detection of *Helicobacter pylori* in cow's milk. Letters in Applied Microbiology. 2002;**35**:504-507

[36] Meng X, Zhang H, Law J, Tsang R, Tsang T. Detection of *Helicobacter pylori* from food sources by a novel multiplex PCR assay. Journal of Food Safety. 2008;**28**(4):609-619

[37] Fernández M, Contreras M, Suárez P, Gueneau P, García-Amado MA. Use of HP selective medium to detect *Helicobacter pylori* associated with other enteric bacteria in seawater and marine molluscs. Letters in Applied Microbiology. 2007;**45**:213-218

[38] Samie A. Prevalence of campylobacter species, helicobacter pylori and Arcobacter species in stool samples from the Venda region, Limpopo, South Africa: Studies using molecular diagnostic methods. Journal of Infection. 2007;**54**:558-566

[39] Jiménez DF. Mediadores Bacterianos de la Inflamacion en La Gastritis. Revista Cubana de Medicina. 1999;**38**:276-283

[40] Grávalos DC, González E. Cancer gastrico. Sociedad Española de Oncología Médica. 2017; pp. 1-16. Available from: https://seom.org/info-sobre-el-cancer/estomago

[41] American Cancer Society. Obtenido de Society, American Cancer Atlanta, Ga: American Cancer. 2016, http://www.cancer.org/cancer-de-estomago-pdf

[42] Hinojosa MM. 2017. Obtenido de: http://www.inen.sld.pe/portal/documentos/pdf/educacion/091115_CANCER%20GASTRICO%20-%20JEMH.pdf

[43] Jiménez DF. Cancer gastrico: Factores de riesgo. Revista Cubana de Oncología. 1998;**14**:171-179

[44] Gisbert J. Infección por Helicobacter pylori. 2016. Obtenido de http://www.aegastro.es/sites/default/files/archivos/ayudas-practicas/19_Infeccion_por_Helicobacter_pylori.pdf

[45] Ofelia CC, Jorge MQ, Harold BG, Alfonso CM, Edson GC, Milagros DM, et al. Prevalencia de helicobacter pylori en pacientes sintomáticos de consulta externa de la red Rebagliati (EsSalud), Lima, Perú, en el período 2010—2013. Revista de Gastroenterología del Perú. 2016;**36**(1):49-55

[46] Scott B. Diagnóstico Microbiológico. Buenos Aires—Argentina: Panamericana; 2009

[47] Secretary of Health Secretaria de Salud. Guia para la aplicacion de pruebas rapidas. Mexico: Printed and Made in Mexico; 2006

[48] Hernández Ramírez D, Cabiedes J. Immunological Techniques that Support the Diagnosis of the Autoimmune Diseases. México D.F, México: Laboratorio de Inmunología, Departamento de Inmunología y Reumatología, Instituto Nacional de Ciencias Médicas y Nutrición Salvador Zubirán; 2010

[49] Siavoshi F, Taghikhani A, Malekzadeh R, Sarrafnejad A, Kashanian M, Jamal AS, et al. The role of mother's oral and vaginal yeasts in transmission of *Helicobacter pylori* to neonates. Archives of Iranian Medicine. 2013;**16**(5):288-294

[50] ad-bio H. pylori Ag Prueba Rápida en Casete (muestras fecales). 2017; Obtenido de: http://www.annardx.com/productos/images/productos/diagnostica/pruebas-rapidas/ad0192c-hpylori-ag-rev-cpdf.pdf

[51] Iglesias G. Tecnicas de biologia molecular. Desde Mendel hasta las moléculas. 2008;1. Obtenido de: https://genmolecular.com/tecnicas-de-biologia-molecular/

[52] Farfan BM. Biologia Molecular Aplicada Al Diagnostico Clinico. Revista Médica Clínica Las Condes. 2015;**26**(6):788-793

[53] Ferrús A. Survival and viability of *Helicobacter pylori* after inoculation into chlorinated drinking water. Water Research. 2007;**41**(15):3490-3496

[54] Pagola MF. Caracterización de la infección por *Helicobacter pylori* en pacientes con úlcera gástrica. Scielo/ Medisur. 2009;**7**(6):3-11

[55] Veenendaal RA, Lichtendahl-Bernards AT, Peña AS, Endtz HP, van Boven CP, Lamers CB. Effect of transport medium and transportation time on culture of *Helicobacter pylori* from gastric biopsy specimens. Journal of Clinical Pathology. 1993;**46**(6):561-563

[56] SCREEN. Test Rapido Antigene. Obtenido de: http://www.screenitalia.it/wp-content/uploads/2017/11/Istruzioni-Screen-H.PyloriSITA-1.pdf

Section 2

Diversity of Tretaments for *H. pylori* Infection Worldwide

Chapter 3

Development of a Novel Antibacterial Medicine that Targets a Characteristic Lipid of the Cell Membranes of *Helicobacter pylori*

Kiyofumi Wanibuchi, Hisashi Masui, Takashi Takahashi and Hirofumi Shimomura

Abstract

Helicobacter pylori is one of the most prevalent causes of gastritis. This pathogen colonizes for many years human stomach and asymptomatically leads the persons to chronic gastritis. The eradication of *H. pylori* from human stomach is, therefore, important in order to prevent the digestive diseases including peptic ulcers and gastric cancer that develop via chronic atrophic gastritis. Wide-spectrum antibiotics such as amoxicillin and metronidazole are used for the treatment for *H. pylori* infectious diseases. However, the *H. pylori* strains resistant to these antibiotics are increasing year by year around the world. On this basis, we need urgently to develop the antibacterial medicines that act on *H. pylori* with a novel mechanism. Recent studies by our group have demonstrated that *H. pylori* shows susceptibility to the bactericidal action of indene compounds derived from decomposition of vitamin D. The bactericidal action of indene compounds is selective not against commonplace bacteria but against *H. pylori*. The indene compounds turned out to target the *H. pylori*'s phosphatidylethanolamine that retains a myristic acid as the saturated fatty acid side chain. These findings will contribute to the development of new antibacterial medicines specialized to the treatment for *H. pylori* infectious diseases.

Keywords: *Helicobacter pylori*, phosphatidylethanolamine, myristic acid, vitamin D, indene compound

1. Introduction

Helicobacter pylori is a Gram-negative microaerophilic helical bacillus equipped with polar flagella as the motility organ. This bacterium colonizes human stomach and causes chronic atrophic gastritis [1]. In addition to gastritis, the patients infected with this pathogen are capable of having various digestive diseases such as gastric ulcer, duodenal ulcer, gastric mucosa-associated lymphoid tissue (MALT) lymphoma, and gastric cancer [2–7]. Therefore, the eradication of *H. pylori* from human stomach is aggressively carried out around the world. Wide-spectrum antibiotics such as amoxicillin, metronidazole, and clarithromycin are used for the treatment for *H. pylori* infectious diseases. However, the *H. pylori* strains resistant to the wide-spectrum antibiotics have been increasing year after year [8]. Especially, almost all *H. pylori* strains clinically isolated from African people have been acquiring the resistance to amoxicillin and metronidazole. In addition, wide-spectrum antibiotics act not only on *H. pylori* but also on commonplace bacteria inhabiting the mucosa of mouth and intestines. Therefore, the patients infected with *H. pylori*, who orally take wide-spectrum antibiotics for the treatment, often suffer from side effects such as stomatitis, constipation, and loose bowels resulted from the collapse of the balance of either oral bacterial flora or enterobacterial flora. When the side effects are serious, the patients develop pseudomembranous colitis accompanied with bloody feces and are compelled to discontinue the eradication of *H. pylori* [9]. To solve the difficult problems on the chemotherapy, we have to develop a novel antibacterial medicine that acts on only *H. pylori* without affecting the survival of human mucosal bacterial flora.

The assimilation of exogenous cholesterol into the cell membranes is one of the unique biological features of *H. pylori*. A part of cholesterol assimilated into the cell membranes is modified with a α-glucose at the carbon position-3 of its steroid framework, and the cholesteryl glucosides generated are used as the bacterial cell membrane constituents [10]. A previous study by our group has revealed that *H. pylori* possesses at least three types of cholesteryl glucosides, cholesteryl-α-D-glucopyranoside (CGL), cholesteryl-6-*O*-tetradecanoyl-α-D-glucopyranoside (CAG), and cholesteryl-6-*O*-phosphatidyl-α-D-glucopyranoside (CPG) (**Figure 1**) [11]. In addition to the three cholesteryl glucosides, other researchers have identified the lyso-type of CPG [12]. CGL is synthesized by the catalytic action of cholesterol α-glucosyltransferase (CGT) that localizes to the cytoplasm-side of the inner membrane of *H. pylori* [13–15]. CGT transfers a glucose derived from a uridine diphosphate glucose (UDP-Glc) to the cholesterol. Although the enzyme proteins involved in the synthesis of either CAG or CPG remain to be clarified, a recent study by other group has demonstrated that the enzymatic activities for the synthesis of CAG and CPG are detected in *H. pylori*'s outer membrane and inner membrane, respectively [16]. In addition, both enzymatic activities for the synthesis of CAG and CPG turned out to use phosphatidylethanolamine (PE) as the substrate [16]. In sum, the CGL acyltransferase (CGLAT) transfers a fatty acid derived from PE to the CGL and thereby synthesizes CAG. Meanwhile, the CGL phosphatidyltransferase (CGLPT) transfers a phosphatidyl group derived from PE to the CGL and thereby synthesizes CPG.

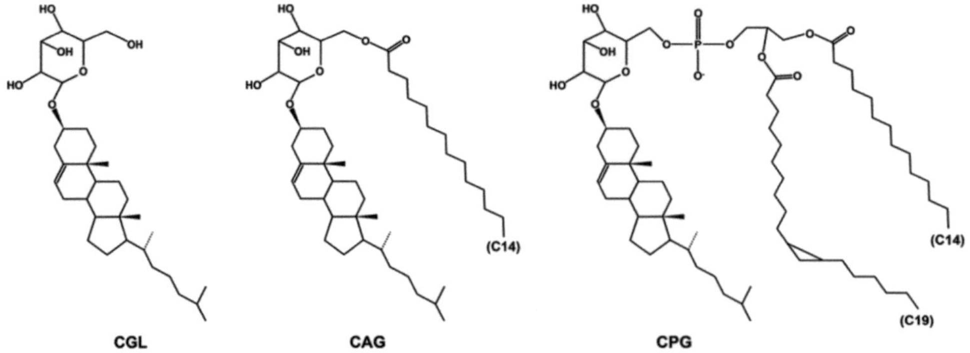

Figure 1.
Chemical structures of cholesteryl glucosides found in H. pylori cell membranes. In addition to the three types of cholesteryl glucosides, H. pylori possesses the lyso-type of CPG that dissociated a myristic acid. CGL, cholesteryl-α-D-glucopyranoside; CAG, cholesteryl-6-O-tetradecanoyl-α-D-glucopyranoside; CPG, cholesteryl-6-O-phosphatidyl-α-D-glucopyranoside; C14, myristic acid; C19, phytomonic acid.

A number of studies, including our own, have revealed that *H. pylori* assimilates exogenous cholesterol in order to acquire the resistance to the antibacterial actions of antibiotics and lipophilic compounds [17–20]. Meanwhile, *H. pylori* glucosylates the assimilated cholesterol to evade the host immune systems and/or to detoxify the toxic steroid compounds with 3β-hydroxyl [12, 21]. The mechanism as for cholesterol uptake of *H. pylori*, however, remained for many years to be clarified. In a study in 2012, it has been revealed that PE of *H. pylori* cell membranes functions as a cholesterol-binding lipid [22]. PE is the most predominant glycerophospholipid component composing Gram-negative bacterial cell membranes. The PE of Gram-negative bacteria such as *Enterobacteriaceae* bacteria and *Pseudomonas aeruginosa* retains a palmitic acid ($C_{16:0}$) as the saturated fatty acid side chain, whereas the PE of *H. pylori* retains a myristic acid ($C_{14:0}$) as the saturated fatty acid side chain [22–26]. In sum, the PE molecular species composition of *H. pylori* turned out to completely differ from that of typical Gram-negative bacteria. A previous study by our group has demonstrated that the PE accounts for greater than 60% in the total lipids (excluding lipopolysaccharide) of *H. pylori* in the logarithmic growth phase [27]. Moreover, it has been revealed that the PE molecular species (DMPE) with two myristic acids accounts for approximately 30% in the total PE molecular species of *H. pylori* [22]. Intriguingly, DMPE showed higher binding affinity for cholesterol than for cholesteryl ester (**Figure 2**). In sum, the selective intermolecular interaction was found between the low-molecular-weight hydrophobic compounds.

Based on a number of studies including our own, the overview from the cholesterol assimilation to the cholesterol glucosylation was partially clarified in *H. pylori*: (1) cholesterol binds at least to DMPE of the outer membrane of *H. pylori* and is assimilated into the membranes; (2) a part of cholesterol is glucosylated by the catalytic action of CGT localized to the cytoplasm-side of the inner membrane, and thereby CGL is generated; (3) CGL is next exchanged to CAG and CPG by the enzymatic actions of CGLAT and CGLPT that localize to the outer membrane and the inner membrane, respectively (**Figure 3**). CGT utilizes an UDP-Glc as the glucose donor of cholesterol. Both enzymes of CGLAT and CGLPT utilize PE (myristoyl-PE) as the acyl group donor and phosphatidyl group donor of CGL,

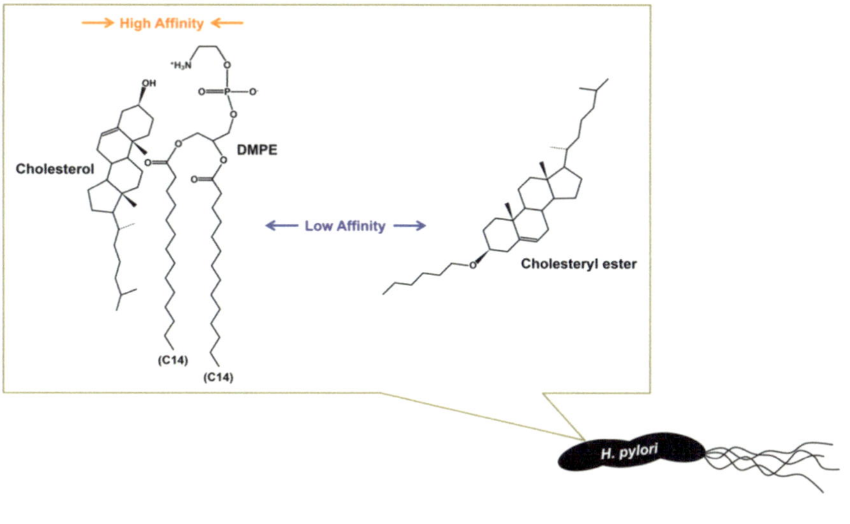

Figure 2.
Binding affinity of dimyristoyl-phosphatidylethanolamine of H. pylori cell membranes for either cholesterol or cholesteryl ester. Dipalmitoyl-PE with two palmitic acids ($C_{16:0}$) shows the high binding affinity for both of cholesterol and cholesteryl ester, whereas dimyristoyl-PE (DMPE) with two myristic acids ($C_{14:0}$) shows the selective high binding affinity only for cholesterol.

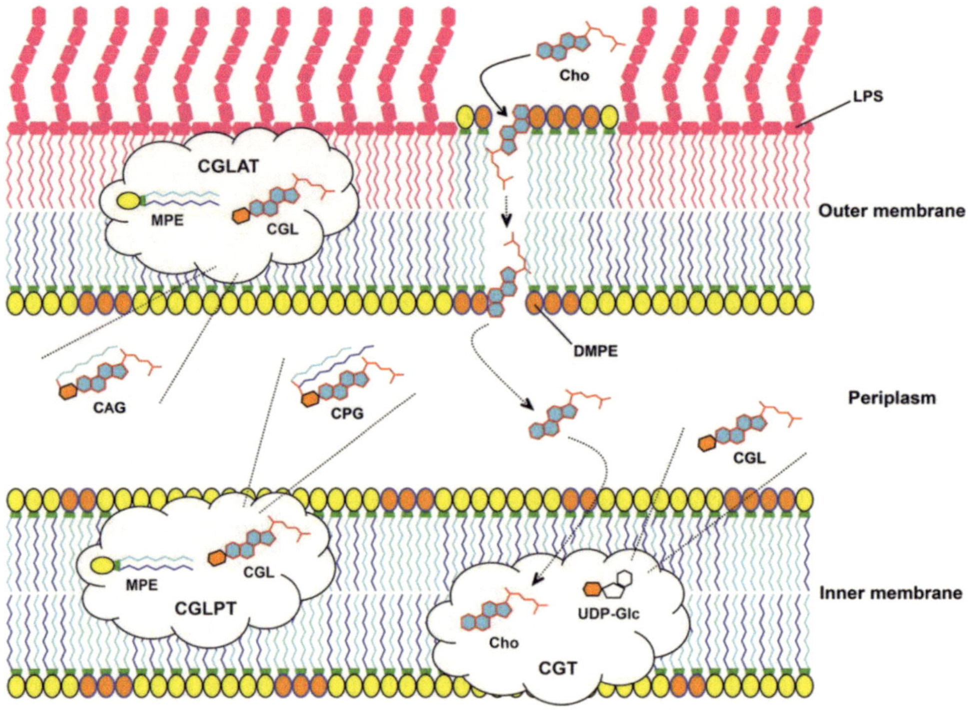

Figure 3.
Cholesteryl glucoside synthesis and its enzyme localization in H. pylori cell membranes. CGT, cholesterol α-glucosyltransferase; CGLAT, CGL acyltransferase; CGLPT, CGL phosphatidyltransferase; Cho, cholesterol; MPE, myristoyl phosphatidylethanolamine; LPS, lipopolysaccharide; UDP-Glc, uridine diphosphate-glucose.

respectively. Incidentally, cholesterol assimilated into *H. pylori* is distributed to both of the inner and outer membranes, whereas cholesteryl glucosides (CGL, CAG, and CPG) synthesized by *H. pylori* predominantly localize to the outer membrane [17].

As described above, it has been revealed that DMPE is one of the most prevalent lipid components of *H. pylori* cell membranes and shows the unique interaction not with cholesteryl ester but with cholesterol. Apart from this, previous studies by our group have demonstrated that a steroid hormone, progesterone acts on the cholesterol-binding site in the *H. pylori* cell membranes and confers the bactericidal action to *H. pylori* [28, 29]. Although it was unclear as for whether the progesterone shows the selective binding affinity for DMPE, this steroid turned out to destabilize the cell membrane structure of *H. pylori* and to ultimately induce the bacteriolysis. These findings drove us to the investigations of the low-molecular-weight hydrophobic compounds that induce the serious structure change to the DMPE molecule through the specific interaction. This chapter mentions the bactericidal activity of the indene compounds against *H. pylori*.

2. Development of new antibacterial medicines for *H. pylori*

2.1 Finding of an indene compound as the anti-*H. pylori* substance

The anti-*H. pylori* activity of various steroidal compounds was investigated. As a consequence, 25-hydroxyvitamin D_3 and 1,25-dihydroxyvitamin D_3 of secosteroids turned out to confer the strong bacteriolytic action to *H. pylori* [30]. However, these vitamin D_3 derivatives conspicuously attenuated their bactericidal activity by the nonbiological degradation (**Table 1**). In contrast, *H. pylori* did not almost

Seco-steroid		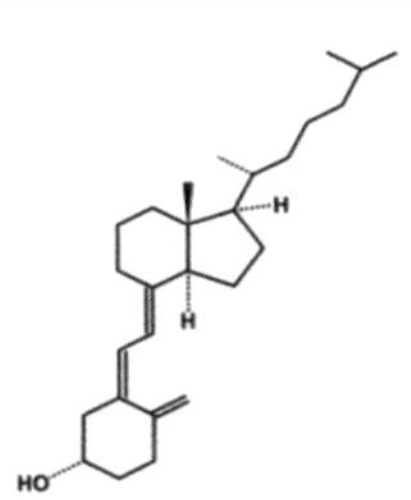 Vitamin D_3	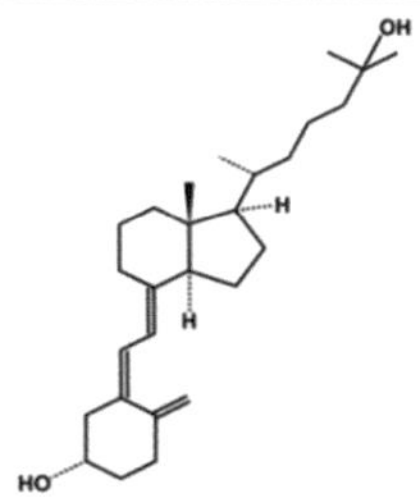 25-hydroxyvitamin D_3	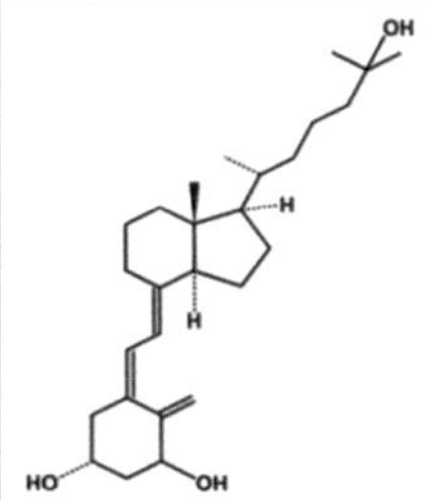 1,25-dihydroxyvitamin D_3
Bactericidal activity	Intact compound	Weak	Strong	Strong
	Degradation	Augmentation	Attenuation	Attenuation

Table 1.
Bacteriolytic action of vitamin D_3 and its derivatives against H. pylori.

succumb to the bacteriolytic action of vitamin D_3. Surprisingly, the nonbiological degradation of vitamin D_3 augmented the bactericidal activity of its secosteroid against *H. pylori*. These results indicated that the vitamin D_3 derivatives directly act as bactericidal substances on *H. pylori*, and that some decomposition product of vitamin D_3 possesses potent bactericidal activity against *H. pylori*. It was, therefore, attempted to extract the anti-*H. pylori* substance from the decomposition products of vitamin D_3. As a consequence, the indene compound species (VDP1), otherwise known as Grundmann's ketone, was successfully obtained [31, 32]. VDP1 is a low-molecular-weight hydrophobic compound in which the indene consisting of 5- and 6-membered rings of hydrocarbons was modified with alkyl, carbonyl, and methyl (**Figure 4**). Intriguingly, *H. pylori* showed high susceptibility to the bacteriolytic action of VDP1, whereas commonplace bacteria such as *Enterobacteriaceae* bacteria, *P. aeruginosa*, and *Staphylococcus aureus* showed insusceptibility to that of VDP1 [30]. In addition, VDP1 conferred the effective bacteriolytic action to *H. pylori* regardless of the assimilation of cholesterol into the cell membranes. These results indicate the possibility that VDP1 is a beneficial fundamental structure for the development of antibacterial medicines to selectively eradicate *H. pylori* without collapsing the balance of human mucosal bacterial flora.

2.2 Interaction between VDP1 and PE molecular species

The collapse induction activity of VDP1 against lipid vesicles was next examined using the unilamellar vesicles prepared with DMPE, dipalmitoyl-PE (DPPE), and dioleoyl-PE (DOPE). Intriguingly, VDP1 turned out to specifically induce the structure collapse of DMPE unilamellar vesicles without affecting the structural stability of either DPPE unilamellar vesicles or DOPE unilamellar vesicles (**Figure 5**). The structure collapse induction activity of VDP1 against DMPE unilamellar vesicles completely corresponded to the bactericidal activity of the indene compound

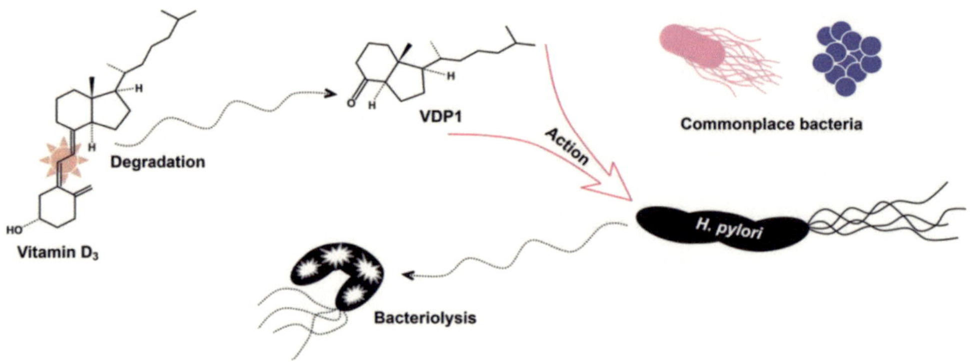

Figure 4.
Bacteriolytic action of VDP1 against H. pylori. H. pylori shows high susceptibility to bacteriolytic action of VDP1 derived from decomposition of vitamin D_3. Meanwhile, commonplace bacteria such as Escherichia coli and Staphylococcus aureus show insusceptibility to bacteriolytic action of VDP1. VDP1, (1R,3aR,7aR)-1-[(1R)-1,5-dimethylhexyl]octahydro-7a-methyl-4H-inden-4-one.

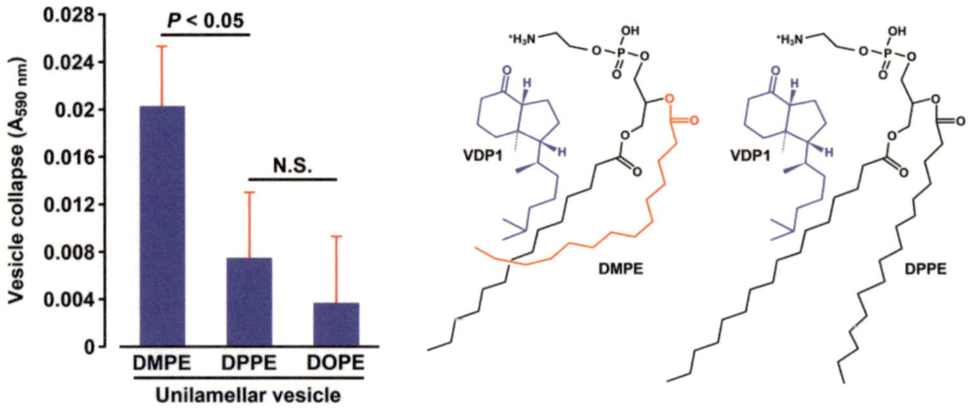

Figure 5.
Specific intermolecular interaction between VDP1 and DMPE. Dye-containing unilamellar vesicles were prepared with DMPE, dipalmitoyl-PE (DPPE) or dioleoyl-PE (DOPE) and incubated for 5 minutes in the presence or absence of VDP1. The absorbance ($A_{590\ nm}$) of dye released from the PE unilamellar vesicles was measured (left graph). The data were obtained from the three independent experiments and are denoted with the mean $A_{590\ nm}$ ± standard deviation. Statistical significance ($P < 0.05$) was calculated by the Student's t-test. N.S. denotes "no statistical significance." VDP1 induces the selective conformation change to the DMPE unilamellar vesicles. The intermolecular interactions between VDP1 and PE molecular species were simulated by the computational chemistry (right panel). VDP1 induces the conformational change only to a myristic acid side chain in the PE molecule without affecting the conformational stability of a palmitic acid side chain in the PE molecule.

against *H. pylori* that abundantly contains DMPE in the cell membranes. Based on these results, VDP1 was considered to specifically interact with the DMPE, to induce the serious structure change to the myristic acid side chain in the PE molecule, and to ultimately disrupt the vesicular conformation of DMPE. In addition, these results strongly suggested that VDP1 exerts the bactericidal effect on *H. pylori* by targeting at least DMPE of the cell membranes.

The intermolecular interaction between VDP1, DMPE, and DPPE was, therefore, simulated by the computational chemistry. One of the computer simulations showed that VDP1 induces "the winding-structure change" to a myristic acid side chain in DMPE molecule, while VDP1 induced no structure change to a palmitic acid side chain in DPPE molecule (**Figure 5**). The alkyl of VDP1 seemed to be crucial conformation for the induction of the structure change of the myristic acid side chain of DMPE. In other words, the slight difference of the length of carbon chain composing the fatty acids in PE molecules appeared to play an important role on the specific interaction between VDP1 and PE molecular species.

2.3 Bactericidal mechanism of the indene compound species

As described earlier, VDP1 was considered to confer the bacteriolytic action to *H. pylori* by the disruption of the cell membranes through the induction of the structure change of DMPE that is one of the most prevalent PE molecular species constructing the bacterial cell membranes. To investigate in detail the crucial conformation of VDP1 for exerting the structure collapse effect on DMPE unilamellar vesicles and for exerting the antibacterial effect on *H. pylori*, various VDP1 derivatives were chemically synthesized [33]. The structure collapse induction activity of VDP1 against DMPE unilamellar vesicles was already ascertained to almost completely correspond to the bactericidal activity of the indene compound against *H. pylori*. When the carbonyl of VDP1 was replaced with a hydroxyl, the indene compound (VD3-1) maintained both activities against DMPE unilamellar vesicles and *H. pylori* (**Table 2**). As seen in VDP1, VD3-1 turned out to confer no structure collapse induction activity against DPPE unilamellar vesicles. In addition, VD3-1 also had no influence on the viability of commonplace bacteria such as *Enterobacteriaceae* bacteria, *P. aeruginosa*, and *S. aureus*. Intriguingly, VD2-2 that lacks the alkyl chain of VD3-1 was ascertained to induce no structure collapses of either DMPE unilamellar vesicles or DPPE unilamellar vesicles and to completely forfeit the effective bactericidal activity against *H. pylori*. In combination with the result of computer simulation as for the intermolecular interaction between VDP1 and DMPE, these results indicate that the alkyl structure in the indene compound

Indene compound	Collapse induction activity		Bactericidal activity		Summary
	DMPE vesicle	DPPE vesicle	*H. pylori*	Others*	
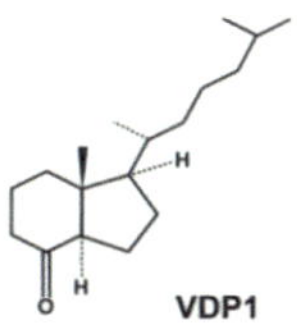 VDP1	Potent	Lack	Potent	Lack	Crucial conformation on the induction of structure change of the myristic acid side-chain in PE molecule 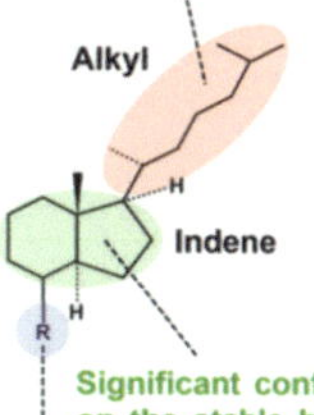 Significant conformation on the stable binding to PE molecule Significant conformation on the reinforcement of electrostatic attraction to the phosphate head of PE molecule R, Carbonyl or Hydroxyl
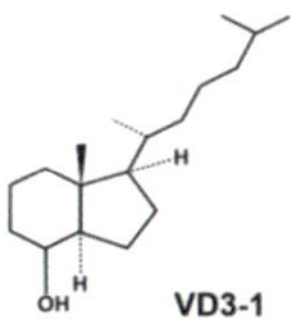 VD3-1	Potent	Lack	Potent	Lack	
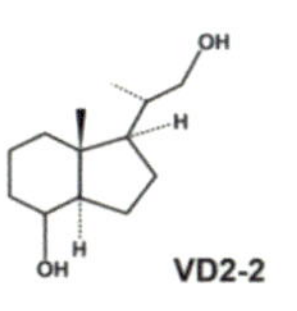 VD2-2	Lack	Lack	Lack	Lack	

Escherichia coli, Klebsiella pneumoniae, Proteus mirabilis, Serratia marcescens, Salmonella sp., Pseudomonas aeruginosa, and Staphylococcus aureus. VD3-1, (1R,3aR,7aR)-7a-methyl-1-((R)-6-methylheptan-2-yl)octahydro-1H-inden-4-ol; VD2-2, (1R,3aR,7aR)-1-((S)-1-hydroxypropan-2-yl)-7a-methyloctahydro-1H-inden-4-ol.

Table 2.
Relationship between indene compounds, PE unilamellar vesicles and H. pylori.

species plays a crucial role on the induction of the structure change of the myristic acid side chain in DMPE molecule. Moreover, the alkyl structure in the indene compound species turned out to be essential for exerting the effective bacteriolytic action to *H. pylori*. The functional groups such as carbonyl and hydroxyl of the indene compound species seem to be significant conformation for bonding to the phosphate head in the PE molecules with an electrostatic attraction. Meanwhile, the indene-ring structure is guessed to be significant to stabilize the hydrophobic interaction between the indene compound species and PE molecules.

A recent study by our group has demonstrated that VDP1 confers the anti-bacterial action not only to *H. pylori* but also to other *Helicobacter* species [33]. Especially, *Helicobacter felis* showed high susceptibility to the bacteriolytic action of VDP1, as similar to *H. pylori*. *H. felis* is a Gram-negative microaerophilic spiral bacillus possessing bipolar tufts of flagella. This bacterium is isolated from the gastric mucosa of cats and dogs [34–36]. As seen in *H. pylori*, *H. felis* causes chronic gastritis and gastric MALT lymphoma in mouse when it colonizes the mouse stomach [37, 38]. An earlier study by our group has revealed that a myristic acid accounts for approximately 16% in the fatty acid composition of *H. felis* PE, and that the PE molecular species retaining a myristic acid and a palmitic acid accounts for approximately 37% in total PE molecular species of the bacteria [39]. Though *H. felis* completely succumbs to the bacteriolytic action at the same concentration of VDP1 (less than 3 μg/ml) that eradicates *H. pylori*, this *Helicobacter* species did not possess DMPE. On this basis, VDP1 is considered to interact not only with DMPE but also with myristoyl-PE that retains a myristic acid as one of the two fatty acid side chains. In addition, *H. felis* turned out to possess lauryl-PE as the most prevalent PE molecular species. The PE molecular species retaining a lauric acid ($C_{12:0}$) and a palmitic acid accounted for approximately 40% in total PE molecular species of *H. felis*. In sum, large parts of PE molecular species of *H. felis* bind a palmitic acid and either a myristic acid or a lauric acid as the fatty acid side chains. Given that a lauric acid is shorter in the length of carbon chain than a myristic acid, we can assume that VDP1 collapses the vesicular conformation consisting not only of myristoyl-PE but also of lauryl-PE. In the future, it will need to elucidate the hydrophobic interaction between VDP1 and lauryl-PE in addition to myristoyl-PE.

In contrast, *Helicobacter cinaedi* showed low susceptibility to the bacteriolytic action of VDP1, even though the PE molecular species composition in *H. cinaedi* is similar to the PE molecular species composition in *H. felis* [39]. *H. cinaedi* is a Gram-negative rod-like bacillus equipped with bipolar flagella and isolated from the intestinal tracts and livers of various mammals such as human, dog, cat, and hamster [40–42]. Therefore, this bacterium is classified into the enterohepatic *Helicobacter* species [43, 44]. Meanwhile, *H. pylori* and *H. felis* are classified into the gastric *Helicobacter* species. Most of the persons infected with *H. cinaedi* have no clinical symptoms, but some persons suffer from systematic inflammations, namely phlegmone, arthritis, and meningitis, due to the bacteremia [45]. Although it is unclear as for why *H. cinaedi* is lower in the VDP1-susceptibility than the two *Helicobacter* species, the involvement of lipopolysaccharide (LPS) is considered as one possibility. LPS is a glycolipid constructed of a long polysaccharide chain and fatty acids and is one of the composition components of the outermost layer of the outer membrane of Gram-negative bacteria [46]. The part of polysaccharide chain in LPS comes into direct contact with the outsides of the bacterial cells and limits the membrane permeability of various lipophilic compounds. The LPS contents in *H. cinaedi* may be higher than those in *H. pylori* and *H. felis*. The membrane permeability of VDP1 through the LPS barrier may be, therefore, stricter in *H. cinaedi* than in *H. pylori* and *H. felis*. Further investigation will be necessary to compare the LPS contents between the *Helicobacter* species.

Based on the current studies, the following bactericidal mechanism of the indene compounds synthetically derived from vitamin D in *H. pylori* was proposed: the indene compounds bind to the myristoyl-PE (including DMPE) of *H. pylori* cell membranes, induce "the winding-structure change" to the myristic acid side chain

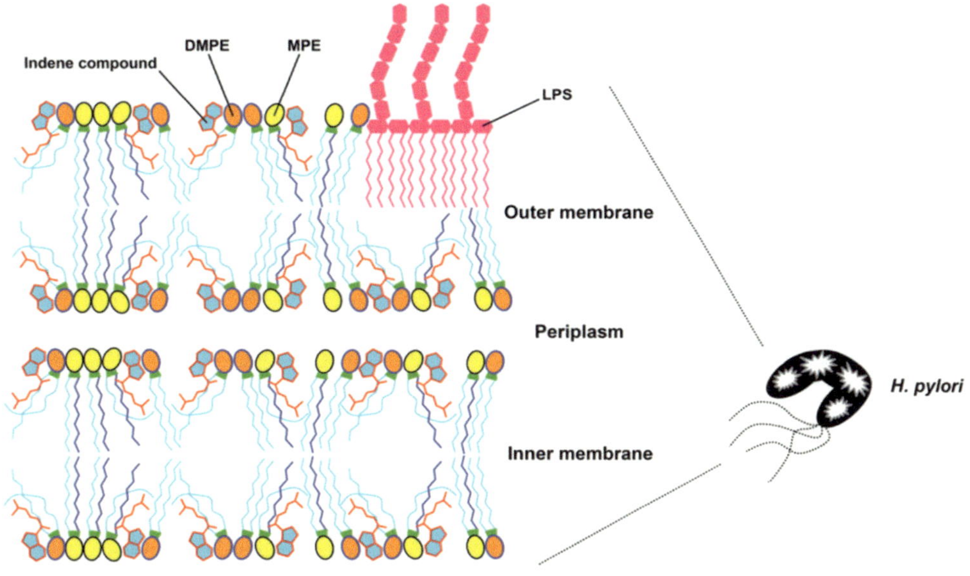

Figure 6.
A proposed bactericidal mechanism of the indene compound species for H. pylori. The indene compound species such as VDP1 and VD3-1 bind to the myristoyl-PE of H. pylori cell membranes and induce "the winding-structure change" to the myristic acid side chain of the especially DMPE. H. pylori ultimately lyses via the destabilization of the membrane conformation.

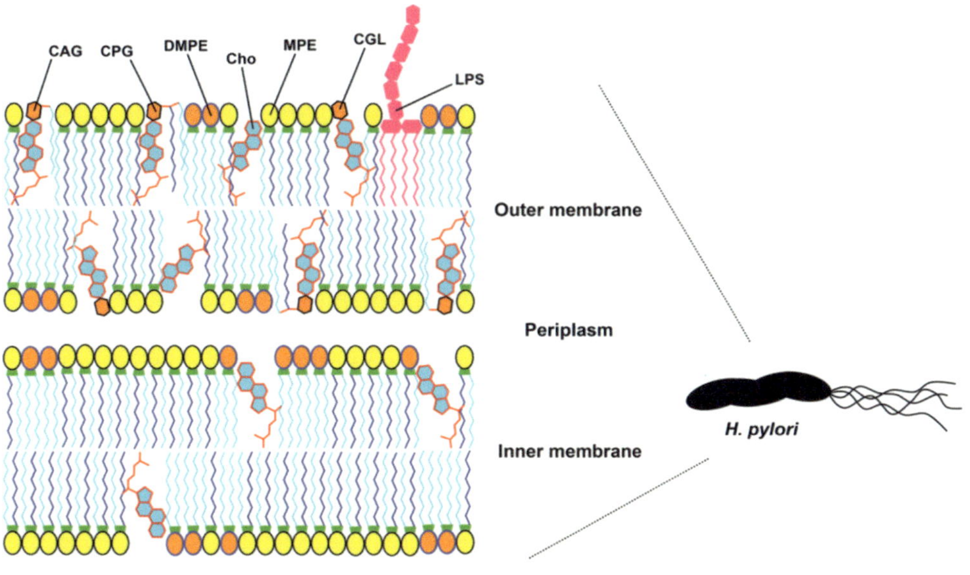

Figure 7.
Role of cholesterol and cholesteryl glucosides in H. pylori. Cholesterol (Cho) binds to the myristoyl-PE (MPE) including dimyristoyl-PE (DMPE) of the H. pylori's cell membranes but has no influence on the stability of the cell membrane conformation. As similar to cholesterol, no cholesteryl glucosides (CGL, CAG, and CPG) affect the cell membrane stability of H. pylori. These steroidal compounds are assimilated as the membrane lipid constituents of H. pylori and serve to strengthen the cell membrane lipid barrier. Incidentally, VDP1 confers the bacteriolytic action to H. pylori regardless of the cholesterol assimilation into the cell membranes.

in the PE molecules, destabilize the membrane conformation, and ultimately confer the bacteriolytic action to *H. pylori* (**Figure 6**).

In the case of the cholesterol assimilation in *H. pylori*, cholesterol is distributed to both membranes of the outer membrane and the inner membrane, and a part of the cholesterol is, thereafter, metabolized to cholesteryl glucosides (CGL, CAG, and CPG), and these metabolites localize to the outer membrane (**Figure 7**). Cholesterol and cholesteryl glucosides have no influence on the stability of the cell membrane conformation of *H. pylori*, and rather these steroidal compounds serve to strengthen the membrane lipid barrier of the bacteria on the limitation of the permeability of lipophilic compounds. A recent study by other group has demonstrated that cholesteryl glucosides are responsible for the morphological maintenance of *H. pylori*, for the acquirement of resistance to antibiotics such as polymyxin B, colistin, and tetracycline, and for the promotion of biofilm formation [47]. This suggests that cholesteryl glucosides of *H. pylori* play an important role to limit the membrane permeability of various low-molecular-weight compounds. However, VDP1 confers the bacteriolytic action even to *H. pylori* retaining cholesterol and cholesteryl glucosides. Further investigation will be necessary to clarify the detailed intermolecular interactions between myristoyl-PE and steroidal compounds.

3. Conclusions

Almost all hydrophobic drugs are pharmacologically designed to inhibit the functions of either protein molecules or nucleic acids in the target creature species. However, no drugs that target a characteristic lipid molecule in the creatures are discovered for many years. In addition, a number of biochemists on lipid research leave great achievements in the analysis of biosynthetic enzymes of various lipophilic compounds such as fatty acids and complex lipids and in the identification of receptors of various hydrophobic ligands such as steroid hormones and eicosanoids. However, these achievements are not as for lipid itself but as for merely proteins. This chapter described the unique interaction between lipids: the indene compound species specifically disrupt the vesicular conformation consisting of DMPE. These findings will bring the new aspects to the drug discovery research and the lipid biochemistry research.

Acknowledgements

This work was supported by a Grant-in-Aid from the Adaptable and Seamless Technology Transfer Program through Target-Driven R&A (A-STEP), JSPS KAKENHI (grant number 15 K08006), and JKA promotion funds from KEIRIN RACE.

Conflict of interest

The authors declare no conflict of interest.

DOI: http://dx.doi.org/10.5772/intechopen.86165

Author details

Kiyofumi Wanibuchi[1], Hisashi Masui[1], Takashi Takahashi[1]
and Hirofumi Shimomura[2]*

1 Faculty of Pharmaceutical Sciences, Yokohama University of Pharmacy, Kanagawa, Japan

2 Independent Researcher, Kumamoto, Japan

*Address all correspondence to: shimomura20090601@gmail.com

References

[1] Marshall B, Warren JR. Unidentified curved bacilli on gastric epithelium in active chronic gastritis. Lancet. 1983;**1**:1273-1274

[2] Graham DY. *Helicobacter pylori*: Its epidemiology and its role in duodenal ulcer disease. Journal of Gastroenterology and Hepatology. 1991;**6**:105-113

[3] Forman D. The Eurogast study group. An international association between *Helicobacter pylori* infection and gastric cancer. Lancet. 1993;**341**:1359-1363

[4] Wotherspoon AC, Oriz-Hidalgo C, Falzon MR, Isaacson PG. *Helicobacter pylori*-associated gastritis and primary B-cell gastric lymphoma. Lancet. 1999;**338**:1175-1176

[5] Uemura N, Okamoto S, Yamamoto S, Matsumura M, Yamaguchi S, Yamakido M, et al. *Helicobacter pylori* infection and the development of gastric cancer. The New England Journal of Medicine. 2001;**345**:829-832

[6] Peek JRM, Blaser MJ. *Helicobacter pylori* and gastrointestinal tract adenocarcinoma. Nature Reviews Cancer. 2002;**2**:28-37

[7] Stolte M, Bayerdorffer E, Morgner A, Alpen B, Wundish T, Thiede C, et al. *Helicobacter* and gastric MALT lymphoma. Gut. 2002;**50**:III19-III24

[8] De Francesco V, Giorgio F, Hassan C, Manes G, Vannella L, Panella C, et al. Worldwide *H. pylori* antibiotic resistance: A systematic review. Journal of Gastrointestinal and Liver Diseases. 2010;**19**:409-414

[9] Trifan A, Girleanu I, Cojocariu C, Sfarti C, Singeap AM, Dorobat C, et al. Pseudomembranous colitis associated with a triple therapy for *Helicobacter pylori* eradication. World Journal of Gastroenterology. 2013;**19**:7476-7479

[10] Shimomura H, Hosoda K, Hirai Y. Interaction of *Helicobacter pylori* cell membrane with non-esterified cholesterol and other steroids. Open Journal of Medical Microbiology. 2013;**3**:70-79

[11] Hirai Y, Haque M, Yoshida T, Yokota K, Yasuda T, Oguma K. Unique cholesteryl glucosides in *Helicobacter pylori*: Composition and structural analysis. Journal of Bacteriology. 1995;**177**:5327-5333

[12] Wunder C, Churin Y, Winau F, Warnecke D, Vieth M, Lindner B, et al. Cholesterol glucosylation promotes immune evasion by *Helicobacter pylori*. Nature Medicine. 2006;**12**:1030-1038

[13] Lebrun AH, Wunder C, Hildebrand J, Churin Y, Zähringer U, Lindner B, et al. Cloning of a cholesterol-α-glucosyltransferase from *Helicobacter pylori*. The Journal of Biological Chemistry. 2006;**281**:27765-27772

[14] Lee H, Wang P, Hoshino H, Ito Y, Kobayashi M, Nakayama J, et al. α1,4-GlcNAc-capped mucin-type *O*-glycan inhibits cholesterol α-glucosyltransferase from *Helicobacter pylori* and suppress *H. pylori* growth. Glycobiology. 2008;**18**:549-558

[15] Hoshino H, Tsuchida A, Kametani K, Mori M, Nishizawa T, Suzuki T, et al. Membrane-associated activation of cholesterol α-glucosyltransferase, an enzyme responsible for biosynthesis of cholesteryl-α-D-glucopyranoside in *Helicobacter pylori* critical for its survival. Journal of Histochemistry and Cytochemistry. 2011;**59**:98-105

[16] Jan HM, Chen YC, Shih YY, Huang YC, Tu Z, Ingle AB, et al. Metabolic labelling of cholesteryl glucosides in *Helicobacter pylori* reveals how the uptake of human lipids enhances bacterial virulence. Chemical Science. 2016;**7**:6208-6216

[17] Shimomura H, Hosoda K, Hayashi S, Yokota K, Oguma K, Hirai Y. Steroids mediate resistance to the bactericidal effect of phosphatidylcholines against *Helicobacter pylori*. FEMS Microbiology Letters. 2009;**301**:84-94

[18] McGee DJ, George AE, Trainor EA, Horton KE, Hildebrandt E, Testerman TL. Cholesterol enhances *Helicobacter pylori* resistance to antibiotics and LL-37. Antimicrobial Agents and Chemotherapy. 2011;**55**:2897-2904

[19] Trainor EA, Horton KE, Savage PE, Testerman TL, McGee DJ. Role of the HefC efflux pump in *Helicobacter pylori* cholesterol-dependent resistance to ceragenins and bile salts. Infection and Immunity. 2011;**79**:88-97

[20] Correia M, Casal S, Vinagre J, Seruca R, Figueiredo C, Touati E, et al. *Helicobacter pylori*'s cholesterol uptake impacts resistance to docosahexanoic acid. International Journal of Medical Microbiology. 2014;**304**:314-320

[21] Shimomura H, Hosoda K, McGee DJ, Hayashi S, Yokota K, Hirai Y. Detoxification of 7-dehydrocholesterol fatal to *Helicobacter pylori* is a novel role of cholesterol glucosylation. Journal of Bacteriology. 2013;**195**:359-367

[22] Shimomura H, Hosoda K, Hayashi S, Yokota K, Hirai Y. Phosphatidylethanolamine of *Helicobacter pylori* functions as a steroid-binding lipid in the assimilation of free cholesterol and 3β-hydroxl steroids into the bacterial cell membrane. Journal of Bacteriology. 2012;**194**:2658-2667

[23] Dunnick JK, O'Leary WM. Correlation of bacterial lipid composition with antibiotic resistance. Journal of Bacteriology. 1970;**101**:892-900

[24] Kearns DB, Robinson J, Shimkets LJ. *Pseudomonas aeruginosa* exhibits directed twitching motility up phosphatidylethanolamine gradients. Journal of Bacteriology. 2001;**183**:763-767

[25] Shokri A, Larsson G. Characterisation of the *Escherichia coli* membrane structure and function during fed batch cultivation. Microbial Cell Factories. 2004;**3**:9

[26] Amine A, Saloua KS, Mouadh M, Alya EIM, Ahmed L. The absence of the "GATC-binding protein SeqA" affects DNA replication in *Salmonella enterica* serovar typhimurium, DNA replication and related cellular processes. In: Kusic-Tisma J, editor. DNA replication and related cellular processes. Rijeka, Croatia: InTech; 2011

[27] Shimomura H, Hayashi S, Yokota K, Oguma K, Hirai Y. Alteration in the composition of cholesteryl glucosides and other lipids in *Helicobacter pylori* undergoing morphological change from spiral to coccoid form. FEMS Microbiology Letters. 2004;**237**:407-413

[28] Hosoda K, Shimomura H, Hayashi S, Yokota K, Hirai Y. Steroid hormones as bactericidal agents to *Helicobacter pylori*. FEMS Microbiology Letters. 2011;**318**:68-75

[29] Amgalanbaatar A, Shimomura H, Hosoda K, Hayashi S, Yokota K, Hirai Y. Antibacterial activity of a novel synthetic progesterone species carrying a linoleic acid molecule against *Helicobacter pylori* and the hormonal effect of its steroid on a murine macrophage-like cell line. The Journal of Steroid Biochemistry and Molecular Biology. 2014;**140**:17-25

[30] Hosoda K, Shimomura H, Wanibuchi K, Masui H, Amgalanbaatar A, Hayashi H, et al. Identification and characterization of a vitamin D_3 decomposition product bactericidal against *Helicobacter pylori*. Scientific Reports. 2015;**5**:8860. DOI: 10.1038/srep08860

[31] Windaus A, Grundmann W. Über die konstitution des vitamin D_2. II. Justus Liebigs Annalen der Chemie. 1936;**524**:295-299

[32] Sicinski RR, DeLuca HF. Ruthenium tetroxide oxidation of Grundmann's ketone derivative from vitamin D_3. Bioorganic and Medical Chemistry Letters. 1995;5:159-162

[33] Wanibuchi K, Hosoda K, Ihara M, Tajiri K, Sakai Y, Masui H, et al. Indene compounds synthetically derived from vitamin D have selective antibacterial action on *Helicobacter pylori*. Lipids. 2018;**53**:393-401

[34] Lee A, Hazell SL, O'Rourke J, Kouprach S. Isolation of a spiral-shaped bacterium from the cat stomach. Infection and Immunity. 1988;**56**:2843-2850

[35] Paster BJ, Lee A, Fox JG, Dewhirst FE, Tordoff LA, Fraser GJ, et al. Phylogeny of *Helicobacter felis* sp. Nov., *Helicobacter musterae*, and related bacteria. International Journal of Systematic Bacteriology. 1991;**41**:31-38

[36] Hansen TK, Hansen PS, Nørgaard A, Nielsen H, Lee A, Andersen LP. *Helicobacter felis* does not stimulate human neutrophil oxidative burst in contrast to '*Gastrospirillum hominis*' and *Helicobacter pylori*. FEMS Immunology and Medical Microbiology. 2001;**30**:187-195

[37] Enno A, O'Rourke JL, Howlett CR, Jack A, Dixon MF, Lee A. MALToma-like lesions in the murine gastric mucosa after long-term infection with *Helicobacter felis*. The American Journal of Pathology. 1995;**147**:217-222

[38] Mohammadi M, Redline R, Nedrud J, Czinn S. Role of the host in pathogenesis of *Helicobacter*-associated gastritis: *H. felis* infection of inbred and congenic mouse strains. Infection and Immunity. 1996;**64**:238-245

[39] Amgalanbaatar A, Hosoda K, Shimomura H. Phosphatidylethanolamine, but not phosphatidylglycerol-cardiolipin, isolated from two species of *Helicobacter* binds cholesterol over cholesteryl ester. Lipids. 2015;**50**:799-804

[40] Kiehlbauch JA, Brenner DJ, Cameron DN, Steigenwalt AG, Makowski JM, Baker CN, et al. Genotypic and phenotypic characterization of *Helicobacter cinaedi* and *Helicobacter fennelliae* strains isolated from human and animals. Journal of Clinical Microbiology. 1995;**33**:2940-2947

[41] Gebhart CJ, Fennell CL, Murtaugh MP, Stamm WE. *Campylobacter cinaedi* is normal intestinal flora in hamsters. Journal of Clinical Microbiology. 1989;**27**:1692-1694

[42] Fox JG, Handt L, Sheppard BJ, Xu S, Dewhirst FE, Motzel S, et al. Isolation of *Helicobacter cinaedi* from the colon, liver, and mesenteric lymph node of a rhesus monkey with chronic colitis and hepatitis. Journal of Clinical Microbiology. 2001;**39**:1580-1585

[43] Mikkonen TP, Kärenlampi RI, Hänninen ML. Phylogenetic analysis of gastric and enterohepatic helicobacter species based on partial HSP60 gene sequences. International Journal of Systematic and Evolutionary Microbiology. 2004;**54**:753-758

[44] Fowsantear W, Argo E, Pattinson C, Cash P. Comparative proteomics of *Helicobacter* species: The discrimination of gastric and enterohepatic *Helicobacter* species. Journal of Proteomics. 2013;**97**:245-255

[45] Kawamura Y, Tomida J, Morita Y, Fujii S, Okamoto T, Akaike T. Clinical and bacteriological characteristics of *Helicobacter cinaedi* infection. Journal of Infection and Chemotherapy. 2014;**20**:517-526

[46] Rietschel ET, Kirikae T, Schade FU, Mamat U, Schmidt G, Loppnow H, et al. Bacterial endotoxin: Molecular relationship of structure to activity and function. The FASEB Journal. 1994;**8**:217-225

[47] Qaria MA, Kumar N, Hussain A, Qumar S, Doddam SN, Sepe LP, et al. Roles of cholesteryl-α-glucoside transferase and cholesteryl glucosides in maintenance of *Helicobacter pylori* morphology, cell wall integrity, and resistance to antibiotics. Molecular Biology and Physiology. 2018;**9**:e01523-e01518

Chapter 4

Pharmacotherapy of Peptic Ulcer Disease and Latest Research

Balaji Ommurugan and Vanishree Rao

Abstract

Peptic ulcers have unquestionably been a disease of the twentieth century. Epidemiological data for this disease and its complications have shown striking variation in incidence and prevalence. Various drugs have been used to treat peptic ulcer disease like proton-pump inhibitors, histamine (H2) receptor antagonists, prostaglandin analogues and sucralfate. Because these drugs are complex, expensive and toxic, efforts have been constantly made to find a suitable, palliative and curative agent for the treatment of peptic ulcer disease from natural products of plant and animal origin. Recently, antioxidants are being used to treat peptic ulcer disease. Antioxidants help in scavenging the free radicals and controlling the oxidative stress responsible for the progression of peptic ulcer.

Keywords: gastritis, gastric ulcers, oxidative stress, antioxidant treatment

1. Introduction

Peptic ulcers have unquestionably been a disease of the twentieth century. Epidemiological data for this disease and its complications have shown striking variation in incidence and prevalence. Peptic ulcer is defined as a local defect or excavation on the surface of the stomach with a mucosal break of diameter 5 mm or larger, usually produced by sloughing of the inflammatory necrotic tissue. Aetiology of peptic ulcer is fiercely debated and is believed that peptic ulcers develop due to imbalance between aggressive factors (*Helicobacter pylori*, non-steroidal anti-inflammatory drugs, gastric acid) and protective factors (mucin, bicarbonate, prostaglandins) leading to interruption of mucosal integrity [1].

The major forms of peptic ulcer include chronic duodenal ulcer, chronic gastric ulcer, Zollinger-Ellison syndrome (ZES), drug-induced ulcers and stress-induced peptic ulcer. Various factors are implicated to play a pivotal role in pathogenesis of ulceration like sedentary life style, alcohol, smoking, spicy food, physiological stress, drugs like non-steroidal anti-inflammatory drugs (NSAIDs) and various bacterial infections [1]. Oxidative stress has emerged as one of the major pathogenic factors in progression of ulcer as it directly impairs the cellular function and promotes cellular organelle damage in mitochondria, lysosomes and nucleus [2].

Stress-induced peptic ulcer is a pathological condition affecting the gastrointestinal tract. Stress ulcers are commonly found in the gastric mucosa anywhere within the stomach to the duodenum. Pathogenesis is mainly due to reduction in mucosal blood flow or a breakdown in other normal mucosal defence mechanisms. Effective therapy remains elusive in the treatment of stress-induced peptic ulcers [3]. One of the common denominators for the occurrence of the disease is involvement of free radicals, an increase in histamine release and decreased mucous production. Reactive oxygen species are generated by various metabolic activities, and antioxidant enzymes like superoxide dismutase, catalase, lipid peroxidase and glutathione peroxidase control their accumulation. Any imbalance in the activity of these enzymes leads to faulty disposal of free radical and their accumulation [4].

Alcohol is one of the leading causes of peptic ulcer disease. The mechanism of ethanol-induced gastric lesions is varied including the depletion of gastric mucus content, damaged mucosal blood flow and mucosal cell injury. It decreases bicarbonate and mucus production by which it produces necrotic lesion in gastric mucosa. Ethanol initiates apoptosis which leads to cell death. It also releases superoxide dismutase and hydroperoxyl free radical species in the biological system [4].

Various drugs have been used to treat peptic ulcer disease like proton-pump inhibitors, histamine (H_2) receptor antagonists, prostaglandin analogues and sucralfate. Because these drugs are complex, expensive and toxic, efforts have been constantly made to find a suitable, palliative and curative agent for the treatment of peptic ulcer disease from natural products of plant and animal origin. Recently antioxidants are being used to treat peptic ulcer disease. Antioxidants help in scavenging the free radicals and controlling the oxidative stress responsible for the progression of peptic ulcer [2]. Coenzyme Q10 (CoQ10) and L-glutamine have antioxidant property, and their role as antioxidants has been documented in the literature in treating medical conditions [5–8].

2. Historical aspect

Gastric acid secretion had always been the topic of debate for the last 100 years with greater emphasis thrown on molecular as well cellular mechanisms involved in gastric acid secretion. Gastric juice was chemically analysed, and hydrochloric acid (HCL) was first isolated from gastric juice in 1824 by William Prout [9]. After the discovery of histamine (H_2) receptor by James Black in 1971, antagonists were available for the treatment of peptic ulcer [10]. After the scintillating discovery of proton-pump inhibitors in 1989, the treatment of peptic ulcer was revolutionized as it blocks the final step of acid synthesis in the stomach lumen.

2.1 Gastric acid regulation

2.1.1 Central regulation

The central nervous system and enteric nervous system play a major role in the regulation of acid secretion along with hormones, paracrine agents as well as second messengers. The acid secretion occurs in three phases, namely, the cephalic, gastric, and intestinal phases [11]. The dorsal motor nucleus of the vagus (DMNV), the nucleus tractus solitarius (NTS) and the hypothalamus play a major role in central regulation of acid secretion. The DMNV plays a crucial role in integrating the sensory input from the hypothalamus and visceral input from the NTS and supplies efferent fibres to the stomach via the vagus, thereby primarily helping in motility rather than secretion. The ventromedial hypothalamus exerts an inhibitory influence on acid secretion with its stimulation causing decreased acid secretion and vice versa [11]. The sensory receptors of the stomach present within the muscle layer as well as mucosa of the stomach help in detecting the mechanical, chemical as well as the thermal stimuli, and these sensory impulses are carried to the central nervous system via sympathetic afferent as well as the vagal nerve fibres [11].

DOI: http://dx.doi.org/10.5772/intechopen.86386

2.1.2 Peripheral mechanism

Intrinsic mechanisms of the stomach regulate acid secretion, and these include neural stimulation via the vagus and gastrin and histamine release from G cells and enterochromaffin-like (ECL) cells, respectively. All these stimuli directly act on the parietal cells. Acetylcholine also helps in the regulation of acid secretion [12]. The histamine released acts on the histamine receptor type 2 (H_2) on the parietal cells, leading to activation of cyclic adenosine monophosphate pathway and calcium-sensitive pathway resulting in stimulation of H^+ K^+-ATPase on parietal cells [13].

2.2 Mechanisms of cytoprotection

The term cytoprotection coined by Robert is defined as protection against gastric mucosal injury by mechanisms other than neutralisation of gastric acid [14]. An explosion of investigations led to the discovery that endogenous prostaglandins are involved in cytoprotection via putative mechanisms which includes mucus secretion, release of bicarbonate, maintenance and strengthening of mucosal blood flow and free radical scavenging [15–18]. The normal gastric mucosa without exogenous insult remains hostile to the acidic milieu of gastric lumen. Gastric mucosal defence can be categorised into pre-epithelial defence which is secretion of mucus gel, epithelial defence with surface epithelial cells withstanding pH <2.5 and the post-epithelial barrier with parietal cells at the base of the gland [19].

2.2.1 Stimulation of mucus and bicarbonate secretion

The mucus barrier is made of mucus, lipids and proteins. These form a continuous gel and along with bicarbonate secretion protect the stomach from acidic insult [20]. Cytoprotective agents like prostaglandins have shown to increase the mucus gel thickness but does not protect the surface epithelium in contrast to protection of the deeper layers [21]. Mucin also helps in reepithelization of mucosa. It was identified that bicarbonate helps in cytoprotection and acts by metabolically dependent process as well as by passive diffusion [22]. Prostaglandins help in increasing the bicarbonate secretion, and bicarbonate in turn forms the mucus bicarbonate barrier [23]. Bicarbonate also directly helps in lowering the hydrogen ion concentration in the gastric mucosa [14].

2.2.2 Strengthening of gastric mucosal barrier

The apical membrane, the so-called tight junctions between the surface epithelial cells, prevents back diffusion of acid and hence forms a major mucosal barrier. Phospholipids on the luminal surface of gastric epithelium form a hydrophobic lining and thereby contribute in preventing the water-soluble hydrogen ions to pass through. Prostaglandins increase concentration of these phospholipids [24].

2.2.3 Regulation of mucosal blood flow

Vascular injuries to sub-epithelial capillaries with increased vascular permeability and circulatory stasis lead to functional impairment of gastric microcirculation. Upregulation of mucosal blood flow maintains oxygenation and nutrient supply. Increase in blood supply to mucosa helps in regulating bicarbonate mediated acid neutralisation and in absorption of injurious agents [25].

2.2.4 Effects on gastric motility

Mucosal compression is said to play an important role in epithelial necrosis and ulceration. Gastric hypercontraction accounts for mucosal compression. The gastric mucosa is protected by the action of circular muscles which causes flattening of gastric mucosal folds, thereby leading to increase in mucosal surface area ultimately reducing volume of irritants coming in contact with the mucosa. Various substances like prostaglandins and mast cell stabilisers aid in this process adding to cytoprotection [26].

2.2.5 Scavenging free radicals

Free radicals cause lipid peroxidation and damage to intracellular components. It leads to ischemia of gastric mucosa, thereby causing severe damage to the mucosa. Vitamin E and selenium are well-known antioxidants shown to have protective effect on stress and chemical-induced gastric lesions [27].

2.2.6 Endogenous mediators on gastric cytoprotection

Prostaglandins, L-cysteine, methionine and epidermal growth factor are said to be cytoprotective. Imbalance between two metabolites of arachidonic pathway is also said to contribute to gastric injury. Literature data suggests prostaglandins help in gastric protection by increasing the gastric blood supply and decreasing the synthesis of leukotrienes, thus playing a significant role in cytoprotection [28]. Therefore, cytoprotection is a multifactorial phenomenon.

2.3 Pathogenesis of peptic ulcer

Peptic ulcers are chronic with ~99% ulcers occurring in the duodenum and stomach with the former being four times higher than the latter [29]. Factors causing peptic ulcers include increased acid secretion, impaired mucosal defence, free radical and lipid peroxidation.

2.3.1 Increased acid secretion

Pepsin activity in gastric juice and acidity of gastric juice are important determinants of ulcer formation. The famous Schwartz's dictum "no acid-no ulcer" becomes accurate when amplified to "no acid and peptic activity", as pepsin contributes to the digestive power of the stomach. This dictum is supported by various therapeutic drugs like antacids and anti-secretory drugs, but much to everyone's anguish, ulcer recurs once therapy is stopped [30].

2.3.2 Impaired mucosal defence

The tight epithelial junctions form a barrier preventing hydrogen ion back diffusion. Recent evidences suggest surface phospholipids form a hydrophobic lining on the gastric epithelium and hence retard the passage of hydrogen ions. NSAIDS and *Helicobacter pylori* infection disrupt the mucosal barrier and are known to increase the diffusion of hydrogen ions [31].

2.3.3 Free radical and peroxidation

Free radical contains unpaired electrons, and it plays an important role in pathogenesis of ischemia/reperfusion injury. Free radicals can nick deoxyribonucleic acid

(DNA) and provoke uncontrolled chain reactions like lipid peroxidation. Acute and chronic gastric ulcers are caused by oxygen-derived free radicals, and in one study, infusion of superoxide-generating system into rat celiac artery-induced gastrointestinal bleeding was shown [32].

2.4 Predisposing factors for peptic ulceration

2.4.1 Helicobacter infection

Helicobacter pylori causes antral gastritis in more than 95% of patients with duodenal ulcer than 75% with gastric ulcer. This organism adheres to the mucosal epithelium close to the gap junctions and releases urea and ammonia producing an alkaline environment with raised pH. This creates an environment for the organism to survive, and release of ammonia is cytotoxic to the gastric cells. Gastric metaplasia occurs, and colonisation of these heterotrophic islands results in mucosal injury and gastric ulceration. Oxidative stress has been implicated in the pathogenesis of *Helicobacter pylori* infections, and increased oxidative damage by *Helicobacter pylori* is responsible for epithelial injury, altered epithelial proliferation and increased apoptosis [33].

2.4.2 Non-steroidal anti-inflammatory drugs

NSAIDs are known to cause various injuries in the gastric tract ranging from haemorrhages and petechiae to erosions with ulcers. These drugs are known to cause mucus glycoprotein denaturation in the stomach and sloughing of epithelial cells. Also, drugs like aspirin causes intracellular protons to accumulate in the parietal cells and leads to localised acid accumulation by the process called back diffusion of acid. These drugs also cause labialization of lysosomes leading to cellular autolytic reactions, inhibition of prostaglandins and mast cell degranulation leading to histamine release, inhibition of glucose oxidation and enzymes involved in anabolic reactions. It also increases the production of free radicals [34].

2.4.3 Cigarette smoking

Healing of ulcers is affected by smoking, and it is a known fact that gastric ulcers occur more frequently in smokers. Various theories are put forward as to why cigarette smoking causes ulcers, and some of them includes stimulation of acid secretion, blood flow alteration to gastric mucosa, induction of bile reflux and reduced prostaglandin synthesis [35].

2.4.4 Psychological stress

The CNS and brain gut axis play an important role in stress ulcerogenesis. Various conditions like shock, sepsis, trauma and neurological disorders are now regarded as multifactorial phenomenon. Various interactions between vascular, mucosal and neurohumoral factors and the autonomic nervous system play a critical role in stress ulcerogenesis. Limbic area plays a pertinent role in modulating acid secretion, motility and blood flow [36].

2.4.5 Alcohol

Ethanol causes cell and plasma membrane damage leading to increased membrane permeability finally causing accumulation of sodium and water. It also causes

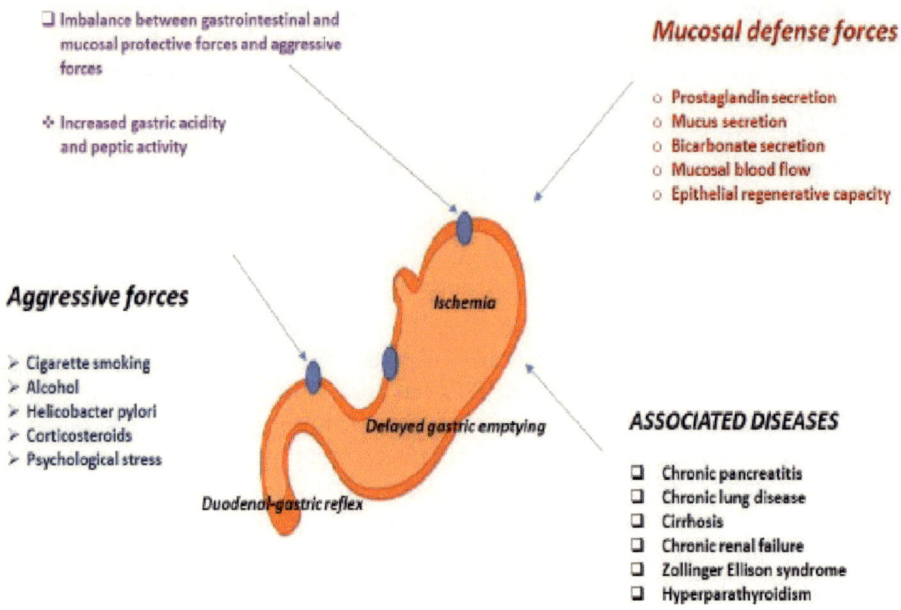

Figure 1.
Pathogenesis of peptic ulcer.

free radical release leading to lipid peroxidation causing gastric lesions. Patients with cirrhosis due to alcohol also have increased incidence of peptic ulcer [37] (**Figure 1**).

2.5 Therapy for acute peptic ulcer

Gastric acid secretion and mucosal defence mechanism have been the target to treat peptic ulcer disease. This has led to discovery of many drugs to treat peptic ulcer disease, and few treatment options have stood the test of time as shown in **Table 1** [38].

2.5.1 H^+/K^+ ATPase inhibitors

It acts by directly blocking the gastric proton pump rather than blocking histamine and cholinergic receptors. There are many drugs available in this class, namely, omeprazole, lansoprazole, rabeprazole and pantoprazole. They block the final step in the acid secretion and thereby have better control over basal as well as nocturnal acid secretion. They are also known to inhibit the growth of *Helicobacter pylor*i [38]. They are now used as first-line agents in the treatment of peptic ulcer, and it has replaced H_2 antagonists.

2.5.2 Prostaglandins

Robert in 1979 showed prostaglandins inhibit gastric acid secretion and help in protection against ulcers caused by NSAIDs, diet, alcohol, smoking and stress. Misoprostol, a prostaglandin analogue, acts by increasing the secretion of mucus as well as bicarbonate, thereby protecting against chronic ulcers. But it helps only in protection against gastric ulcer and not against duodenal ulcers [39]. It is contraindicated in pregnancy due to its abortifacient property. Enprostil, rioprostil and arbaprostil are other known compounds. Other drugs in clinical trials are noclo-prost, enisoprost and mexiprost [39].

DOI: http://dx.doi.org/10.5772/intechopen.86386

Class of drugs	Mechanisms	Use
H2 receptor antagonists (cimetidine, ranitidine, famotidine, nizatidine, roxatidine)	Acid inhibition	*H. pylori*-negative peptic ulcer; replaced by PPI because of inferiority in acid suppression
PPI (omeprazole, pantoprazole, lansoprazole, rabeprazole, esomeprazole)	Most potent acid inhibition	Standard treatment for all *H. pylori*-negative peptic ulcers; prevention of NSAID or aspirin ulcers; essential component in eradication regimen; given intravenously in bleeding ulcers
Prostaglandin analogues (misoprostol*)	Increase mucosal resistance; weak acid inhibition	*H. pylori*-negative gastric ulcer; prevention of NSAID ulcers
***H. pylori* eradication regimens** (PPI plus two antibiotics)	Cure of *H. pylori* infection	Standard therapy in all *H. pylori*-positive ulcers
Bismuth salts (subcitrate, subsalicylate)	Weak antibacterial effect; increase of mucosal prostaglandin synthesis	In quadruple therapy for *H. pylori* eradication

PPI = proton-pump inhibitor, NSAID = non-steroidal anti-inflammatory drug *Contraindicated in pregnancy*

Table 1.
Class of drugs with effect on healing of peptic ulcer.

2.5.3 H_2 receptor antagonists

These drugs act by blocking the H_2 receptor and thereby reduce the release of gastric acid. It is very helpful in reducing 90% of the basal, food-stimulated and nocturnal secretion of gastric acid as well. Literature evidence says it also helps in prevention of stress-induced gastric ulcers. They are used in combination with antacids in the treatment of stress-induced ulcers. These drugs include mainly ranitidine, cimetidine, famotidine and nizatidine. One of the major drawbacks is long duration of administration for ulcer therapy, and recurrence of ulcer after healing is a frequent complication [40].

2.5.4 Muscarinic receptor antagonists

Pirenzepine has more cytoprotective effects when compared with histamine receptor antagonists. It helps in protection against gastric mucosal lesions induced by alcohol, sodium hydroxide (NAOH) and taurocholate. It exerts its action via inhibition of muscarinic (M_1) receptor present in the stomach and reduces basal as well as stimulated acid secretion [41].

2.5.5 Mucosal coating agents

Sucralfate is a basic sulphated disaccharide with aluminium sulphate complex. It helps in forming an adherent coating at the mucosal sites which are ulcerated. It acts by reducing pepsin activity, adsorbs bile salts and acts as barrier to hydrogen ion diffusion. It also binds to both epidermal growth factor (EGF) and fibroblast growth factor (FGF) and helps in enhancing ulcer healing. It is found effective in *Helicobacter pylori* infection [42].

3. Coenzyme Q10

Morton in 1955 in Liverpool identified a quinone-like substance with an ultraviolet absorption at 272 nm from intestinal mucosa of horses and named it as ubiquinone.

Crane and his colleagues in the University of Wisconsin isolated quinone in lipid extracts of mitochondria and named it coenzyme Q because of its unique role in cellular metabolism and energy production. Ernster, a Swedish scientist, expanded the benefits of this molecule as an antioxidant and free radical scavenger. Coenzyme Q10 also plays a major proton-motive role in the energy transfer systems [43].

Coenzyme Q10 is an active quinone with a benzoquinone ring along with 10 isoprenoid side chains. It is structurally related to vitamin K and vitamin E. Naturally it is orange in colour without odour and taste with a molecular weight of 863.34 g/mol. It is stable at temperatures below 46°C. CoQ10 is the prevalent form in humans in contrast to CoQ9 in rats and Q6, Q7 and Q8 in yeast and bacteria. It exists in three forms, the fully oxidised ubiquinone; semiquinone, the free radical form; and ubiquinol, the reduced form [44].

CoQ10 is found in every cell of the human body, mainly located in the phospholipid bilayer of various membranes. It is found in higher concentrations in the heart, liver, muscles and pancreas, which have high energy requirements. It is derived from tyrosine with several vitamins and trace elements as cofactors. Because of this complex biosynthesis, human enzyme and protein defects may cause deficiency of CoQ10 in infants as well as adults. Cellular functions depend on production of adenosine triphosphate (ATP) in mitochondria making electron and proton transfer functions of quinone ring very important in all life forms [43].

Coenzyme Q10 is usually absorbed from the small intestine, and bioavailability depends on the type of preparation and on the route of administration. Evidence says it is absorbed orally with almost 178% increase in serum levels. Some studies also say it is absorbed very minimally due to its lipophilic nature and huge molecular weight. Oil-based preparations of CoQ10 have better absorption [44].

It plays a vital role as intermediate in mitochondrial electron transport chain. CoQ10, an endogenously synthesised lipid-soluble antioxidant along with alpha-tocopherol, acts in scavenging the free radicals generated in the inner mitochondrial membrane. CoQ10 also prevents lipid peroxidation in cells depleted of alpha-tocopherol. It helps in protection of DNA from free radical injury, in recycling of antioxidants such as tocopherol and ascorbate with additional role in cell signalling and gene expression. A direct evidence for the antioxidant property of CoQ10 is shown in literature, where luminescence is eliminated from free radicals when skin cream containing coenzyme Q10 is applied demonstrating the elimination of free radicals by CoQ10. It also helps in maintaining cellular respiration and ATP synthesis. It also helps in decreasing calcium overload in tissues by indirectly stabilising calcium channels [45].

CoQ_{10} deficiencies are due to autosomal recessive mutations, mitochondrial diseases, ageing-related oxidative stress, carcinogenesis processes and also treatment with statins. Many neurodegenerative disorders, diabetes, cancer and muscular and cardiovascular diseases have been associated with low CoQ_{10} levels as well as different ataxias and encephalomyopathies [45, 46]. CoQ10 is generally very well tolerated at doses not exceeding 500 mg. Gastrointestinal (digestive) distress is reported with doses up to 3000 mg daily [45]. Recent evidence also says coenzyme Q10 is used in treatment of peptic ulcer. Few animal studies have tried the use of coenzyme Q10; in one study, indomethacin-induced ulcer in Wistar rats was treated using coenzyme Q10, and favourable results were obtained [47]. CoQ10-mediated gastroprotective effect involves preservation of microvascular permeability, elevation of prostaglandin E_2, improvement of redox status as well as boosting of nitric oxide.

4. Glutamine

Glutamine is one of the 20 amino acids encoded by standard genetic code. It is considered a conditionally essential amino acid. Its side chain is an amide formed by replacing hydroxyl side chain of glutamic acid. In humans, blood glutamine is the most abundant free amino acid, with concentration of about 500–900 μmol/L. It is mainly helpful in protein synthesis, acid base balance, cellular energy (next to glucose), nitrogen donation for anabolic process, carbon donation in citric acid cycle and ammonia transporter in blood circulation. It is produced by enzyme glutamine synthetase from glutamate/ammonia in muscles. Almost 90% of glutamine is synthesized in the muscles [48]. Consumers are cells of the intestine, kidney cells and immune/cancer cells. It is used in cachexia, to reduce infections and to control gut leak after surgery. It also increased intestinal barrier and intestinal permeability. As a preferred substrate for enterocytes, glutamine has shown to support the normal immunological structure and function of the gastrointestinal tract. In animal studies glutamine deprivation is associated with loss of intestinal epithelial integrity, while glutamine supplementation decreases gastrointestinal tract mucosal atrophy. Glutamine also restored ATP levels and reduces cell apoptosis. It is very important during stress and catabolic conditions [49]. So far only one animal study has evaluated the use of L-glutamine in aspirin-induced peptic ulcer model. They found out the L-glutamine was effective in protecting against aspirin-induced gastric lesions in rats [50]. L-Glutamine, commonly used in sports medicine for muscle recovery, has gained medical importance because of its antioxidant properties [51]. The antioxidant properties of L-glutamine has been claimed to be useful in the treatment of peptic ulcer disease in animal studies as well as in very few human studies. Only a few animal studies have been done so far to investigate the role of L-glutamine in the treatment of *Helicobacter pylori* infections, and it was found to be positive, yet human trials have not been done in large [52, 53].

4.1 Ulcer induction methods

Clinical ulcers are usually chronic and are penetrating lesions in comparison with experimentally induced lesions which are acute non-penetrating ulcers healing at faster rates without scar formation. Even though experimental lesions have some limitation, it is still possible to evaluate the therapeutic agents rapidly with reasonable predictability for their therapeutic use. There are various animal models used for evaluating gastric ulcers, and some of the most important will be described below.

Criteria for experimental ulcers proposed by Lee and Bianchi are as follows [54]:

1. It should be simple and easily reproducible with easy quantification of results.

2. Variety of animal species should be made use of.

3. Ulcer should be produced in characteristic sites like the stomach and the first part of the duodenum.

4. Models should include different mechanisms by which ulcers are produced.

5. There should not be any spontaneous healing of ulcers during the observation period.

The various methods available are discussed in the next subsections.

4.1.1 Pylorus ligated rat

Ulcers produced by this method are also called as Shay ulcers as it was first demonstrated by Shay in 1945. In this model, the animals are usually housed in individual cages and fasted for 36 h before ligating the pylorus. The abdomen is opened after anesthetising the rats by a small midline incision just below the xiphoid process. Then the pyloric part of the stomach is ligated without compromising its vascularity. Later the abdomen is closed in layers using interrupted sutures. The animal is made to starve completely without water and is sacrificed after 19 h. The stomach is then dissected out, and the contents of the stomach are used to determine the pH, volume of gastric juice and free and total acidity. The stomach is then cut open along the greater curvature and examined for ulceration. Circular lesions and linear lesions are observed. This model usually has a greater predictive value for antiulcer agents though ulcers in this model are usually localised in the ruminal area of the stomach in comparison to human ulcers which are usually located in the glandular portion of the stomach and duodenal region [55].

4.1.2 Stress ulcers

These ulcers are usually produced by subjecting any species to different types of stress. This model is very easy as it is devoid of any experimental surgery and usage of anaesthesia. It mainly involves the central nervous system, and produced lesions are located in the glandular portion of the stomach.

5. Restraint ulcers

This method was first used by Brodie and Hansen in 1960. Rats are usually fasted for 36 h before the experiment. Later each rat is placed in a piece of galvanised steel window screen of appropriate size. The screen is then moulded around each rat and is held together with wire staples. The animals are made immobile by tightening the limbs together. The test drug is administered 30 min before subjecting the animals to restraint. After 24 h the animals are sacrificed, and their stomach is dissected out along the greater curvature and is subjected to assessment. One drawback of this method was the ulcers were not deep as they did not penetrate the muscularis mucosa and penetrating ulcers were not produced. Some commonly used modifications of this method to overcome the drawbacks include water immersion-induced restraint ulcer, cold and restraint ulcer, swimming stress ulcers and also stress with concurrent administration of NSAIDs and also haemorrhagic shock-induced gastric ulcers in rats [56].

5.1 NSAID-induced gastric mucosal damage

The routinely used drug for experimental induction of ulcers includes diclofenac, ibuprofen, indomethacin, phenylbutazone and aspirin. Usually the test agents are administered 30 min–1 h before the noxious challenge. Later after 4 h the animals are sacrificed and examined for mucosal lesions in the stomach [57].

5.1.1 Histamine-induced gastric ulcers

The vasospastic and the gastric secretion increases shown via the histamine receptors attribute to ulcer formation in this model. It was first described in 1947 in guinea pigs. It was noted that in this model 100% ulceration was produced with notable increase in volume of gastric secretion as well as increment in free and total acidity. Usually the animals are fasted for 36 h, and ulcers are induced by injecting 1 ml of histamine acid phosphate (50 mg base) via intraperitoneal route. Histamine toxicity to animals are prevented using promethazine hydrochloride

5 mg intraperitoneally 15 min prior to and 15 min after histamine administration, respectively. The investigational drug is usually administered 45 min before injecting histamine. After 4 h the animals are sacrificed; and assessment of the stomach is done after dissection, and various indices are calculated [58].

5.1.2 Acetic acid-induced chronic gastric ulcers

Acetic acid at a concentration of 1–30% is used, and usually 0.05 ml per rat is used. It is injected to the submucosal layer of the stomach, penetrating ulcers usually produced can be noted with gross examination, and ulcers are mostly confined by adhesion to contiguous organs. It can be successfully used to screen new antiulcer agents [59].

5.1.3 Serotonin-induced gastric ulcers

Wilhelmi, Wedinger and Veraguth described this method in Wistar rats. Usually rats are fasted for 24 h, and later serotonin creatinine sulphate is dissolved in saline and injected subcutaneously into rats. Usually serotonin is used at a dose of 20 mg/kg, and with this dose, moderate gastric lesions are noted [60].

5.1.4 Ethanol-induced gastric ulcers.

Eighty percent of ethanol in a dose of 5 ml/kg of body weight is usually given orally to the albino rats. If administered intraperitoneally, 40% of ethanol is given, and usually animals are observed for a period of 7–14 days [61].

6. Conclusion

Peptic ulcer being a global problem proper treatment is warranted. Proper screening of *Helicobacter pylori* and ruling out other possible causes could benefit the patient in getting cured with the correct treatment. The latest research proves oxidative stress as one of the major contributing factors for peptic ulcer disease, so the use of antioxidants as a potential agent is highly warranted. Further clinical trials can be done to elicit the efficacy of these antioxidants as potential anti-peptic ulcer drugs.

Author details

Balaji Ommurugan[1*] and Vanishree Rao[2]

1 Drug Safety Physician, Bioclinica Private Limited, India

2 Research Scholar, Mcops, Manipal Academy of Higher Education, India

*Address all correspondence to: puntermmc@gmail.com

References

[1] Prabhu V, Shivani A. An overview of history, pathogenesis and treatment of perforated peptic ulcer disease with evaluation of prognostic scoring in adults. Annals of Medical and Health Sciences Research. 2014;**4**(1):22-29

[2] Tandon R, Khanna RD, Dorababu M, Goel RK. Oxidative stress and antioxidants status in peptic ulcer and gastric carcinoma. Indian Journal of Physiology and Pharmacology. 2004;**48**(1):115-118

[3] Das D, Bandyopadhyay D, Bhattacharjee M, Banerjee RK. Hydroxyl radical is the major causative factor in stress-induced gastric ulceration. Free Radical Biology and Medicine. 1997;**23**(1):8-18

[4] Ko JK, Cho CH. Alcohol drinking and cigarette smoking: A "partner" for gastric ulceration. Chinese Medical Journal; Free China ed. 2000;**63**(12):845-854

[5] Denny N, Chapple IL, Matthews JB. Antioxidant, and anti-inflammatory effects of coenzyme Q10: A preliminary study. Journal of Dental Research. 1999;**78**(543):00008

[6] Heyland DK, Elke G, Cook D, Berger MM, Wischmeyer PE, Albert M, et al. Glutamine and antioxidants in the critically ill patient: A post hoc analysis of a large-scale randomized trial. Journal of Parenteral and Enteral Nutrition. 2015;**39**(4):401-409

[7] Okabe S, Ohtsu K, Takeuch K, Takhal K. Effect of L-glutamine on indomethacin induced gastric lesions in the rat. The Japanese Journal of Pharmacology. 1974;**24**:169-171

[8] Karkaya K, Barut F, Hanci V, Can M, Comert M, Ucan HB, et al. Gastroprotective effects of CoQ10 on ethanol-induced acute gastric lesions. Bratislavské Lekárske Listy. 2015;**116**(1):51-56

[9] Heinz E, Öbrink KJ. Acid formation and acidity control in the stomach. Physiological Reviews. 1954;**34**(4):643-673

[10] Angus JA, Black JW. The interaction of choline esters, vagal stimulation, and H2-receptor blockade on acid secretion in vitro. European Journal of Pharmacology. 1982;**80**(2-3):217-224

[11] Hersey SJ, Sachs G. Gastric acid secretion. Physiological Reviews. 1995;**75**(1):155-190

[12] Goldschmiedt M, Feldman M. Gastric secretion in health and disease. In: Sleisenger MH, editor. Gastrointestinal Disease. Philadelphia: WB Saunders Company; 1993. pp. 521-544

[13] Soll AH. Pathogenesis of peptic ulcer and implications for therapy. New England Journal of Medicine. 1990;**322**(13):909-916

[14] Robert A, Nezamis JE, Lancaster C, Hanchar AJ. Cytoprotection by prostaglandins in rats. Gastroenterology. 1979;**77**(3):433-443

[15] Lacy ER, Ito S. Microscopic analysis of ethanol damage to rat gastric mucosa after treatment with a prostaglandin. Gastroenterology. 1982;**83**(3):619-625

[16] Szabo S, Szelenyi I. Cytoprotection'in gastrointestinal pharmacology. Trends in Pharmacological Sciences. 1987;**8**(4):149-154

[17] Schmidt KL, Miller TA. Morphological characteristics of prostaglandin cytoprotection. Toxicologic Pathology. 1988;**16**(2):223-236

[18] Soll AH, Weinstein WM, Kurata J, McCarthy D. Nonsteroidal anti-inflammatory drugs and peptic

ulcer disease. Annals of Internal Medicine. 1991;**114**(4):307-319

[19] Sanders MJ, Ayalon A, Roll M, Soll AH. The apical surface of canine chief cell monolayers resists H+ back-diffusion. Nature. 1985;**313**(5997):52-54

[20] Younan F, Pearson J, Allen A, Venables C. Changes in the structure of the mucous gel on the mucosal surface of the stomach in association with peptic ulcer disease. Gastroenterology. 1982;**82**(5):827-831

[21] Bickel M, Kauffman GL. Gastric gel mucus thickness: Effect of distention, 16,16-dimethyl prostaglandin E2, and carbenoxolone. Gastroenterology. 1981;**80**(4):770-775

[22] Rees WD, Turnberg LA. Mechanisms of gastric mucosal protection: A role for the 'mucus-bicarbonate' barrier. Clinical Science. 1982;**62**(4):343-348

[23] Allen A, Garner A. Mucus and bicarbonate secretion in the stomach and their possible role in mucosal protection. Gut. 1980;**21**(3):249

[24] Fromm D. Gastric mucosal "barrier". Gastroenterology. 1979;**77**(2):396-398

[25] Pihan G, Rogers C, Szabo S. Vascular injury in acute gastric mucosal damage. Digestive Diseases and Sciences. 1988;**33**(5):625-632

[26] Takeuchi K, Nobuhara Y. Inhibition of gastric motor activity by 16,16-dimethyl prostaglandin E 2. Digestive Diseases and Sciences. 1985;**30**(12):1181-1188

[27] Itoh M, Guth PH. Role of oxygen-derived free radicals in hemorrhagic shock-induced gastric lesions in the rat. Gastroenterology. 1985;**88**(5):1162-1167

[28] Peskar BM, Hoppe U, Lange K, Peskar BA. Effect of nonsteroidal anti-inflammatory drugs (NSAID) on rat gastric leukotriene formation. Gastroenterology. 1987;**92**(5):1573-1573

[29] Desai JK, Goyal RK, Parmar NS. Pathogenesis of peptic ulcer disease and current trends in therapy. Indian Journal of Physiology and Pharmacology. 1997;**41**(1):3-15

[30] Du Plessis DJ. Pathogenesis of gastric ulceration. The Lancet. 1965;**285**(7393):974-978

[31] Isenberg JI, Selling JA, Hogan DL, Koss MA. Impaired proximal duodenal mucosal bicarbonate secretion in patients with duodenal ulcer. New England Journal of Medicine. 1987;**316**(7):374-379

[32] Demir S, Yilmaz M, Koseoglu M, Akalin N, Aslan D, Aydin A. Role of free radicals in peptic ulcer and gastritis. Turkish Journal of Gastroenterology. 2003;**14**(1):39-43

[33] Kuipers EJ, Thijs JC, Festen HP. The prevalence of *Helicobacter pylori* in peptic ulcer disease. Alimentary Pharmacology & Therapeutics. 1995;**9**:59-69

[34] Huang JQ, Sridhar S, Hunt RH. Role of *Helicobacter pylori* infection and non-steroidal anti-inflammatory drugs in peptic-ulcer disease: A meta-analysis. The Lancet. 2002;**359**(9300):14-22

[35] Kurata JH, Nogawa AN. Meta-analysis of risk factors for peptic ulcer: Nonsteroidal antiinflammatory drugs, *Helicobacter pylori*, and smoking. Journal of Clinical Gastroenterology. 1997;**24**(1):2-17

[36] Levenstein S, Ackerman S, Kiecolt-Glaser JK, Dubois A. Stress and peptic ulcer disease. JAMA. 1999;**281**(1):10-11

[37] Friedman GD, Siegelaub AB, Seltzer CC. Cigarettes, alcohol, coffee

and peptic ulcer. New England Journal of Medicine. 1974;**290**(9):469-473

[38] Malfertheiner P, Chan FK, McColl KE. Peptic ulcer disease. The Lancet. 2009;**374**(9699):1449-1461

[39] Freston JW. Overview of medical therapy of peptic ulcer disease. Gastroenterology Clinics of North America. 1990;**19**(1):121-140

[40] Nash J, Lambert L, Deakin M. Histamine H2-receptor antagonists in peptic ulcer disease. Drugs. 1994;**47**(6):862-871

[41] Giorgi-Conciato M, Daniotti S, Ferrari PA, Gaetani M, Petrin G, Sala P, et al. Efficacy and safety of pirenzepine in peptic ulcer and in non-ulcerous gastroduodenal diseases. A multicentre controlled clinical trial. Scandinavian Journal of Gastroenterology. Supplement. 1982;**81**:1

[42] Guth PH. Mucosal coating agents and other non-anti-secretory agents. Digestive Diseases and Sciences. 1987;**32**(6):647-654

[43] Crane FL. Discovery of ubiquinone (coenzyme Q) and an overview of function. Mitochondrion. 2007;7:S2-S7

[44] Bhagavan HN, Chopra RK. Coenzyme Q10: Absorption, tissue uptake, metabolism and pharmacokinetics. Free Radical Research. 2006;**40**(5):445-453

[45] Overvad K, Diamant B, Holm L, Holmer G, Mortensen SA, Stender S. Coenzyme Q10 in health and disease. European Journal of Clinical Nutrition. 1999;**53**(10):764-770

[46] Shults CW. Coenzyme Q10 in neurodegenerative diseases. Current Medicinal Chemistry. 2003;**10**(19):1917-1921

[47] Malash AM, Abdallah DM, Agha AM, Kenawy SA. Gastroprotective efficacy of coenzyme Q10 in indomethacin-induced gastropathy: Other potential mechanisms. Ulcers. 2012;**6**:2012

[48] Miller AL. Therapeutic considerations of L-glutamine: A review of the literature. Alternative Medicine Review: A Journal of Clinical Therapeutic. 1999 Aug;**4**(4):239-248

[49] Novak F, Heyland DK, Avenell A, Drover JW, Su X. Glutamine supplementation in serious illness: A systematic review of the evidence. Critical Care Medicine. 2002;**30**(9):2022-2029

[50] Okabe S, Takeuchi K, Nakamura K, Takagi K. Inhibitory effects of L-glutamine on the aspirin-induced gastric lesions in the rat. Journal of Pharmacy and Pharmacology. 1974;**26**(8):605-611

[51] Heyland DK, Dhaliwal R, Day AG, Muscedere J, Drover J, Suchner U, et al. Reducing deaths due to oxidative stress (The REDOXS© Study): Rationale and study design for a randomized trial of glutamine and antioxidant supplementation in critically-ill patients. Proceedings of the Nutrition Society. 2006;**65**(3):250-263

[52] Hagen SJ, Ohtani M, Zhou JR, Taylor NS, Rickman BH, Blackburn GL, et al. Inflammation and foveolar hyperplasia are reduced by supplemental dietary glutamine during *Helicobacter pylori* infection in mice. The Journal of Nutrition. 2009;**139**(5):912-918

[53] Amagase K, Nakamura E, Endo T, Hayashi S, Hasumura M, Uneyama H, et al. New frontiers in gut nutrient sensor research: Prophylactic effect of glutamine against *Helicobacter pylori*-induced gastric diseases in Mongolian gerbils. Journal of Pharmacological Sciences. 2010;**112**(1):25-32

[54] Lee YH, Bianchi RG. Use of experimental peptic ulcer models for drug screening. Peptic Ulcer. 1971:329-348

[55] Shay H. A simple method for the uniform production of gastric ulceration in rat. Gastroenterology. 1945;**5**:43-61

[56] Levine RJ. A method for rapid production of stress ulcers in rats. In: Peptic Ulcer. Copenhagen: Munksgaard; 1971. pp. 92-97

[57] Djahanguiri B. The production of acute gastric ulceration by indomethacin in the rat. Scandinavian Journal of Gastroenterology. 1968;**4**(3):265-267

[58] Hay LJ, Varco RL, Code CF, Wangensteen OH. The experimental production of gastric and duodenal ulcers in laboratory animals by the intramuscular injection of histamine in beeswax. Surgery, Gynecology & Obstetrics. 1942;**75**:170-182

[59] Okabe S, Pfeiffer CJ. Chronicity of acetic acid ulcer in the rat stomach. Digestive Diseases and Sciences. 1972;**17**(7):619-629

[60] LePard KJ, Stephens RL. Serotonin inhibits gastric acid secretion through a 5-hydroxytryptamine1-like receptor in the rat. Journal of Pharmacology and Experimental Therapeutics. 1994;**270**(3):1139-1144

[61] Oates PJ, Hakkinen JP. Studies on the mechanism of ethanol-induced gastric damage in rats. Gastroenterology. 1988;**94**(1):10-21

Chapter 5

Gastritis Treated by Chinese Medicine

Xiaomei Wang, Guang Ji and Huangan Wu

Abstract

Chronic gastritis is one of the common diseases of the digestive system characterized by many uncomfortable clinical symptoms, and the patient with chronic gastritis has a lower quality of life. Chinese medicine is a branch of medicine in the world, and it has special theory; different methods have been used to treat gastritis for more than 1000 years. We aimed to introduce the special theory and the different methods of Chinese medicine and about its syndrome classification, syndrome differentiation and treatment, diagnosis and treatment process, and criterion of therapeutic effect of chronic gastritis. The mechanism of Chinese medicine on chronic gastritis needs further research.

Keywords: gastritis, Chinese medicine, diagnosis, syndrome classification, syndrome differentiation, treatment

1. Introduction

Chronic gastritis is one of the common diseases of the digestive system and a chronic inflammatory reaction of gastric mucosa caused by several factors, such as *Helicobacter pylori* infection, alcoholism, smoking, stress conditions, and the use of some conventional medicines such as some anti-inflammatory drugs; the infection of *Helicobacter pylori* is its main cause [1, 2]. Chronic non-atrophic gastritis, atrophic gastritis (atrophy, intestinal metaplasia), dysplasia, and carcinogenesis may occur after *Helicobacter pylori* infection [3, 4].

Chronic gastritis is usually divided into chronic superficial gastritis and chronic atrophic gastritis. Chronic superficial gastritis is characterized by no obviously pathological changes. Its common symptoms are abdominal discomfort after eating, dull pain, accompanying belching, and pantothenic acid. Chronic atrophic gastritis is characterized by atrophy and decrease of gastric mucosal epithelium and glands, thinness of gastric mucosa, thickening of the mucosal base, or metaplasia of pyloric gland and intestinal gland or atypical hyperplasia. Chronic atrophic gastritis occurs in approximately 2% of the general population in the United States [5], particularly those older than 60 years and with higher prevalence in females [5, 6], and a Swedish study reported an increased incidence in the population aged between 35 and 45 years [6]. The common symptoms of chronic gastritis are a dull pain in the upper abdomen, abdominal fullness and distention, belching, inappetence, or being thin and anemic. The symptoms of gastritis are easy to relapse which seriously affect their quality of life. Chronic atrophic gastritis with intestinal metaplasia and intraepithelial neoplasia increases the risk of gastric cancer, and more attention has been paid to gastritis clinically.

Traditional Chinese medicine (TCM) has accumulated many years of clinical experience in the diagnosis and treatment of this disease. In 2009, spleen-stomach disease branch of China Association of Chinese Medicine (CACM) organized and formulated the "consensus opinions on TCM diagnosis and treatment of chronic superficial gastritis" and "consensus opinions on TCM diagnosis and treatment of chronic atrophic gastritis," which played a normative role in the diagnosis and treatment of chronic gastritis. In recent years, there are a lot of progress of TCM in the diagnosis and treatment of chronic gastritis. It is necessary to update the consensus opinions to meet clinical needs and better guide clinical work.

Based on the principles of evidence-based medicine, team members of spleen-stomach disease branch of CACM extensively collected evidence-based information, and they successively organized domestic experts of spleen and stomach diseases to summarize and discuss a series of key issues such as syndrome classification, syndrome differentiation and treatment, diagnosis and treatment process, and criterion of therapeutic effect for chronic gastritis. Based on an expert opinion, three rounds of voting followed under internationally accepted Delphi law, the drafting group has fully discussed, revised, and approved the consensus in 2017 (Consensus opinions of TCM diagnosis and treatment experts on chronic gastritis, 2017 edition) [7].

2. TCM diagnosis of chronic gastritis

TCM diagnosis of chronic gastritis is mainly based on symptom diagnosis. Patients with stomachache as the main symptom were diagnosed as "epigastric pain," and patients with epigastric distention as the main symptom were diagnosed as "distention and fullness." If the symptoms of stomachache or epigastric distention are not obvious, it can be diagnosed as "acid regurgitation," "hubbub," and other diseases according to the main symptoms [8, 9].

3. Diagnosis of chronic gastritis by western medicine

The diagnosis of chronic gastritis mainly depends on endoscopy and pathological examination, especially the latter is of greater value. The etiology of chronic gastritis should be determined as far as possible, and endoscopic diagnosis of special gastritis must combine etiology and pathology [10].

3.1 Clinical manifestations

Chronic gastritis is a chronic inflammatory reaction of the gastric mucosa, and most patients with chronic gastritis may have no obvious clinical symptoms. Patients with symptoms mainly manifested a non-specific dyspepsia, such as discomfort in the upper abdomen, fullness, pain, loss of appetite, belching, acid regurgitation, etc. A part also can have forgetfulness, anxiety, depression, and other psychological symptoms [8–10]. There was no significant correlation between the presence and severity of dyspepsia and the histological findings and endoscopic grading of chronic gastritis [8–10].

3.2 Endoscopic and pathological examination

Endoscopic diagnosis: For non-atrophic gastritis, endoscopic examination showed the basic manifestations of mucosal erythema, mucosal hemorrhagic spots or plaques, rough mucosa with or without edema, hyperemia, and exudation. For atrophic gastritis, endoscopic examination showed that the mucosa was red and white, mainly white, with folds flattened or even disappeared. Some mucosal vessels were exposed, which may be accompanied by mucosal granules or nodules. It is described as atrophic gastritis or non-atrophic gastritis with bile reflux, erosion and mucosal bleeding, etc.

Histopathologic diagnosis: Two or more biopsy tissues can be selected as required. The endoscopic physician should provide the site of sampling, endoscopic examination results, and brief medical history to the pathology department. The pathological changes should be reported in each biopsy specimen in each biopsy specimen, such as the grade of *Helicobacter pylori* infection, chronic inflammatory response, activity, atrophy, intestinal metaplasia, and dysplasia (intraepithelial neoplasia). Chronic gastritis biopsy shows atrophy of the inherent glands (including metaplasia atrophy and non-metaplasia atrophy), which can be diagnosed as atrophic gastritis, regardless of the number and degree of atrophy of the biopsy specimen. The clinician may combine the pathological result and the endoscopic view, making the lesion scope and the degree judgment [10].

3.3 Lab examination

Helicobacter pylori is the most important cause of chronic gastritis. Routine detection is recommended. Vitamin B12 and autoantibodies are recommended for diagnosis of atrophic gastritis. Serum gastrin G17, pepsin I and II may help determine whether gastric mucosa atrophy and atrophy [10].

4. Etiology and pathogenesis of chronic gastritis

4.1 Etiology

The stomach is physiologically harmonious, but pathologically it is sluggish [11]. This disease is mainly related to the weakness of spleen and stomach, emotional disorders, improper diet, drugs, exogenous pathogens (*Helicobacter pylori* infection), and other factors; the above factors damage the spleen and stomach, resulting in transport and loss of division, rise and fall disorders, and the occurrence of Qi stagnation, wet resistance, cold coagulation, fire depression, blood stasis, etc., manifested as stomachache, bloating, and other symptoms.

4.2 Disease location

Chronic gastritis is located in the stomach and is closely related to the liver and spleen in TCM theory.

4.3 Pathogenesis

The pathogenesis of chronic gastritis can be divided into two aspects: deficient essential and excessive superficial. This deficiency is mainly manifested as qi (Yang) deficiency and stomach yin deficiency. The main manifestations of excessive superficial are stagnation of qi, dampness and heat, and blood stasis. Spleen deficiency and qi stagnation are the basic pathogenesis of chronic gastritis.

4.4 Change of pathogenesis

The syndrome differentiation of chronic gastritis should examine the evidence and seek the cause. The pathogenesis is related to the specific clinical type. In general, it is often clinically manifested as the syndrome of the combination of the original and the false and the real [8, 9]. In the early stage, the patients were mainly positivistic, while the patients who had been ill for a long time became the deficiency syndrome or the mixture of deficiency and reality. Chronic non-atrophic gastritis is characterized by weakness of the spleen and stomach and disharmony of the liver and stomach [12]. Chronic atrophic gastritis is characterized by weakness of the spleen and stomach, qi stagnation, and blood stasis [13, 14]. Chronic gastritis with bile reflux is more common with disharmony between the liver and stomach [15]. Spleen and stomach dampness-heat syndrome is common in patients with *Helicobacter pylori* infection [16, 17]. For patients with precancerous lesions, qi and yin deficiency, qi stagnation and blood stasis, and damp-heat internal obstruction syndromes are common [18, 19].

5. Syndrome differentiation type of chronic gastritis

Combined with existing consensus and standards, quantitative literature statistical methods were used to conduct statistics on the relatively common clinical single syndromes. The common syndromes were identified as the syndrome of liver-stomach disharmony which includes the syndrome of liver-stomach qi stagnation and the syndrome of liver-stomach heat retention, the syndrome of damp-heat of the spleen and stomach, the syndrome of spleen-stomach weakness including the syndrome of spleen-stomach qi deficiency and the syndrome of spleen-stomach cold syndrome, the syndrome of deficiency of stomach yin, and the syndrome of obstruction of stomach collaterals. The above syndromes can appear alone or in combination, and the clinical diagnosis should be based on the identification of single syndromes.

5.1 Standard of syndrome differentiation

5.1.1 Syndrome of liver-stomach disharmony

5.1.1.1 Syndrome of liver-stomach qi stagnation

Main symptoms are full or painful epigastric distention, distension, or pain in the flanks. Minor symptoms are induced or exacerbated by emotional factors and frequent belching. Symptoms in the tongue and pulse include pink tongue, thin and white moss, and wiry pulse.

5.1.1.2 Syndrome of liver-stomach heat retention

Main symptoms are epigastric burning pain, distension, or pain in the flanks. Minor symptoms are upset and irritability, acid reflux, dry mouth, bitter mouth, and dry stool. Symptoms in the tongue and pulse include red tongue, yellow moss, wiry pulse, or rapid pulse.

5.1.2 Syndrome of damp-heat of the spleen and stomach

Main symptoms are distention and fullness of stomach and abdomen, trapped and heavy body, and loose or sticky stool. Minor symptoms include eating less, anorexia, bitter mouth, bad breath, and drowsy mental. Symptoms in the tongue and pulse include red tongue, yellow and greasy moss, slippery pulse, or rapid pulse.

5.1.3 Weakness of the spleen and stomach

5.1.3.1 Syndrome of spleen-stomach qi deficiency

Main symptoms are epigastric distension or faint stomachache, postprandial aggravation, tired, and weak. Minor symptoms are indigestion and loss of appetite, cold limbs, and thin and sloppy stool. Symptoms in the tongue and pulse include pale tongue or tooth marks, thin and white moss, and weak pulse.

5.1.3.2 Syndrome of deficiency of the spleen and stomach

The main symptom is dull and insistent stomachache, preferring warmth and pressure. Minor disease: stomachache attack or aggravation after fatigue or take cold, spit water, mental fatigue, limb lassitude, diarrhea or with indigestible food. Symptoms in the tongue and pulse include pale and fat tongue with tooth mark, white and slippery moss, and deep and weak pulse.

5.1.4 Syndrome of deficiency of stomach yin

Major symptoms include epigastric burning pain and noise in the stomach. Minor symptoms include hunger and not wanting to eat, dry mouth, and dry stool. Symptoms in the tongue and pulse include red tongue and little saliva, no or little moss, and thin or rapid pulse.

5.1.5 Syndrome of stomach collateral stasis

Main symptoms are fullness in the stomach or pain with definite location. Minor symptoms are stomach pain for a long time and sting pain. Symptoms in the tongue and pulse include dark red tongue or petechiae, ecchymosis, and wiry and unsmooth pulse.

Syndrome diagnosis: with two main symptoms and two minor symptoms, the diagnosis can be made by referring to tongue and pulse.

5.2 Microscopic syndrome differentiation of chronic gastritis

Gastroscope is a tool to observe the color, texture, secretion, peristalsis of gastric mucosa, and mucosal blood vessels to identify the type of syndrome differentiation. Syndrome differentiation under gastroscopy has certain clinical value, especially for patients with no clinical symptoms or poor efficacy after long-term treatment. The classification standards of microscopic syndrome differentiation are as follows [20].

5.2.1 Syndrome of disharmony between liver and stomach

Syndromes are acute and active inflammatory reaction in gastric mucosa, or with bile reflux, gastric peristalsis faster.

5.2.2 Syndrome of spleen-stomach dampness and heat

Syndromes are congestion and edema in gastric mucosa and obvious erosion of thick and turbid mucus.

5.2.3 Syndrome of spleen-stomach weakness

Syndromes include pale gastric mucosa, thinning mucosa, thin and more mucus or mucosal edema, visible submucosal blood vessels, and decreased gastric motility.

5.2.4 Syndrome of stomach yin deficiency

Syndromes are rough mucosal surface, thin and brittle, less secretion, thinner or disappeared plica, fissure-like changes, or visible small vascular network under the mucous membrane.

5.2.5 Syndrome of stomach collateral stasis

Syndromes are granular or nodular gastric mucosa, with intramucosal hemorrhage; gray or brown mucus; visible vascular network; and dark red vascular veins.

6. Clinical treatment of chronic gastritis

The main aim to treat chronic gastritis with traditional Chinese medicine focuses on improving the symptoms and quality of life of the patients and paying close attention to the lesions of erosion and atrophy of gastric mucosa, intestinal metaplasia, and intraepithelial neoplasia (dysplasia).

6.1 Therapeutic principles

The main therapeutic methods of TCM for chronic gastritis include medication, acupuncture, moxibustion therapy, etc. In clinic, appropriate treatment methods can be selected according to the specific situation and combined with dietary adjustment, psychological counseling, and other methods of comprehensive treatment. In the course of treatment, etiologic factors based on differentiation and treatment based on syndrome differentiation should be determined.

6.2 Treatment based on syndrome differentiation

6.2.1 Syndrome of disharmony between the liver and stomach

6.2.1.1 Syndrome of qi stagnation between the liver and stomach

The therapeutic principle is to soothe the liver to smoothen qi and harmonize the stomach. Main prescription includes Chaihu Shugan powder (*Jingyue Quanshu*). Chinese herbal medicine include Bupleurum, tangerine peel, *Fructus aurantii*, peony, *Rhizoma cyperi*, *Ligusticum striatum*, and liquorice. Patient with epigastric pain can add Sichuan neem seed and *Rhizoma corydalis*. Patient with apparent belch can add agarwood and inula flower.

6.2.1.2 Syndrome of heat stagnation in the liver and stomach

Treatment includes cooling the liver and soothing the stomach. Main prescription includes Huagan decoctum (*Jingyue Quanshu*) and Zuo Jin Wan (*Danxi Xinfa*). Medication includes Pericarpium citri reticulatae viride, tangerine peel, white peony root, peony peel, Gardenia, *Alisma*, fritillary bulb of Zhejiang, *Rhizoma coptidis*, and *Evodia officinalis*. Patient with obvious acid reflux can add squid bone and concha arcae. Patient with fullness and discomfort in the chest and hypochondrium can add Bupleurum and Radix curcumae.

6.2.2 Syndrome of damp-heat in the spleen and stomach

Treatment includes clearing heat and removing dampness. Main prescription includes the soup of Huanglian Wendan (Discrimination of Six Causes). Chinese herbal medicine include *Pinellia ternata*, orange peel, *Poria cocos*, immature bitter orange, bamboo shavings, *Rhizoma coptidis*, jujube, and liquorice. Patient with abdominal distension can add *Magnolia officinalis* and betel nut. Patient with belching acid decay can add radish seed, Divine comedy, and hawthorn.

6.2.3 Syndrome of deficiency of the spleen and stomach

6.2.3.1 Syndrome of the spleen and stomach qi deficiency

Treatment includes reinforcing qi to strengthen the spleen. Main prescription includes Xiangsha Liujunzi decoction (*Ancient and Modern Famous Medical Prescription*). Chinese herbal medicine includes costustoot, orange peel, *Pinellia ternata*, *Codonopsis*, *Atractylodes*, *Poria cocos*, and liquorice. Patient with fullness and distention can add citron. Patient with shortness of breath and sweating can add Radix Astragali Preparata. Patient with cold limbs can add cassia twig and *Angelica*.

6.2.3.2 Syndrome of deficiency and cold in spleen and stomach

Treatment includes warming and strengthening the spleen. Prescription includes Huangqi Jianzhong decoction (*Synopsis of the Golden Chamber*) and Lizhong decoction (*Treatise on Febrile Diseases*). Chinese herbal medicines include *Astragalus*, peony, cassia twig, ginger, jujube, maltose, *Codonopsis*, white *Atractylodes rhizome*, dried ginger, and liquorice. Patient with loose stool can add cannon ginger charcoal and fried coix seed. Patient with obvious chills can add aconite.

6.2.4 Syndrome of yin deficiency of stomach

Treatment includes nourishing yin, benefiting the stomach. The main prescription is Yiguan Decoction (*Xu Mingyi Lei'an*). Chinese herbal medicines include radix ginseng, Radix ophiopogonis, Rehmanniae, *Angelica sinensis*, *Fructus lycii*, and Szechwan Chinaberry fruit. Patient with obvious stomachache can add *Paeonia lactiflora* and liquorice. Patient with constipation can add snake gourd fruit and semen cannabis.

6.2.5 Syndrome of stomach collaterals stasis

The treatment includes activating blood circulation and removing blood stasis. Main prescription includes Shixiao powder (*Taiping Huimin Heji Jufang*) and Danshen decoction (*Shifang Gekuo*). Chinese herbal medicines include Wuling zhi, Typhae pollen, *Salvia miltiorrhiza*, Sandalwood, and *Amomum*. Patient with obvious pain can add *Rhizoma corydalis* and *Radix curcumae*. Patient who has shortness of breath and is weak can add *Astragalus* and *Codonopsis*. For patients with complex clinical symptoms and multiple syndromes, the combination of prescriptions corresponding to the pathogenesis can improve the treatment effect. For example, if the pathogenesis of gastritis patient is the deficiency of the spleen and stomach and the disharmony between the liver and stomach, the main prescription should be Xiangsha Liujunzi decoction and Bupleurum Shugan powder.

6.3 Treatment based on disease differentiation

Treating chronic gastritis by disease differentiation is an important part of TCM clinical practice. The principle is to formulate the prescription based on the understanding of the basic pathogenesis of chronic gastritis and then prescribe the prescription according to the syndrome. From the composition of clinical prescriptions, most of them are composed of single syndrome prescriptions. For those without obvious clinical symptoms, treatment can be carried out based on disease differentiation combined with the syndrome differentiation results of the tongue and pulse and gastric mucosa manifestation under endoscope.

In chronic gastritis patients with positive *Helicobacter pylori*, eradication of *Helicobacter pylori* is necessary if there are obvious clinical symptoms or accompanied by atrophy, erosion, intestinal metaplasia, intraepithelial neoplasia, or family history of gastric cancer [8, 10]. The eradication of *Helicobacter pylori* guidelines and drug regimen were need.

Based on the syndrome differentiation, when chronic gastritis is accompanied by gastric mucosa congestion and erosion, Notoginseng powder, *Rhizoma bletillae* powder, and Pearl powder can be added for treatment, and it can be taken with decoction or with warm water after making a paste and taken on an empty stomach. For patients with intramucosal hemorrhage, the herbs to remove blood stasis and stop bleeding can be added, such as *Panax notoginseng* powder and *Rhizoma bletillae* powder. For chronic gastritis patient with precancerous lesions and syndrome of non-spleen-stomach deficient cold can add *Hedyotis diffusa*, *Scutellariae barbatae*, and Chinese lobelia into the compound prescription or use the herbs for promoting circulation and removing stasis, such as *Salvia miltiorrhiza*, *Panax notoginseng*, and Zedoary turmeric.

6.4 Commonly used Chinese patent medicine

6.4.1 Qizhi Weitong granules

It can smooth liver qi and harmonize the stomach to alleviate stomachache. It was usually used for patients with depression or irritability, sigh, belching, chest stuffiness and fullness, and epigastric pain.

6.4.2 Weishu granules

It can regulate qi and eliminate distension and alleviate stomachache. It was usually used for patients with epigastric pain caused by qi stagnation with epigastric distension pain, which extends to two sides, pain relief after belching or flatus, pain aggravation after emotional depression and anger, eating less food, chest distress, and poor defecation.

6.4.3 Wenweishu capsule

It can nourish the stomach and promote Qi circulation to relieve pain. It was usually used for patients with stomachache caused by deficiency and cold in the middle Jiao with epigastric cold pain, abdominal distension and belching, poor appetite, less food, intolerance of cold, and weakness.

6.4.4 Xuhan Weitong granule

It can tonify Qi and the spleen and warm the stomach to relieve pain. It is usually used for patients with stomachache caused by deficiency of the spleen and stomach. The symptoms are epigastric dull pain, tolerance of warmth and pressure, aggravation after catch cold, eating cold food, or stomach empty.

6.4.5 Jianwei Xiaoshi oral liquid

It can tonify the stomach and improves digestion. It was usually used for patients with dyspepsia caused by deficiency of the spleen and stomach. The symptoms are dyspepsia, belching, putrid belching and acid swallowing, abdominal fullness, and distention.

6.4.6 Yangweishu capsule

It can nourish the yin and stomach. It was usually used for patients with epigastric burning pain caused by deficiency of the yin and stomach. The further symptoms are dull pain, feverishness in palms and soles, dry mouth, bitter mouth, poor appetite, and emaciation.

6.4.7 Cubeb Weitong granules

It can activate Qi to promote blood circulation and harmonize stomach to relieve pain. It was usually used for epigastric distension and pricking pain caused by Qi stagnation and blood stasis.

6.4.8 Molodan (concentrated pills)

It can harmonize the stomach and calms the adverse-rising energy, strengthens the spleen to relieve distension and dredge collateral to relieve pain. It was usually used for patients with symptoms of stomachache, fullness, stuffy, indigestion, and loss of appetite and belching.

6.4.9 Wei Fuchun capsule

It can strengthen the spleen and nourish qi and promote blood circulation and detoxification. It was usually used for patients with the precancerous lesions of gastric cancer of chronic atrophic gastritis or adjuvant treatment after gastric cancer surgery.

6.4.10 Dalitong granules

It can clear heat and relieve depression, regulate the stomach and calm the adverse-rising energy, and eliminate stagnation. It was usually used for patients with epigastric fullness and distention syndrome caused by heat stagnation of the liver and stomach. The symptoms include epigastric distension and fullness, belching, poor appetite, heartburn in the stomach, noisy pantothenic acid, epigastric pain, and dry and bitter mouth. The dyskinetic type of functional dyspepsia seen above symptoms.

6.4.11 Weitai granules

It can promote Qi circulation and relieve stomachache. It is usually used for patients with stomachache caused by qi stagnation and blood stasis and dampness and heat stasis. The symptoms are abdominal dull pain, fullness, sour regurgitation, nausea, and vomiting; the discomfort is lessened after eating.

6.4.12 *Jin Weitai capsule*

It can promote qi circulation and relieve pain in the stomach. It is usually used for patients with acute and chronic gastroenteritis, ulcer in the stomach and duodenum caused by qi stagnation of the liver and stomach or dampness and heat stasis.

6.4.13 *Weikang capsule*

It can promote Qi circulation and invigorate the stomach, remove blood stasis and hemostasis, and relieve hyperacidity and pain. It is usually used for patients with epigastric pain caused by Qi stagnation and blood stasis. The further symptoms are pain fixation, acid swallowing noise, and gastric and duodenal ulcers.

6.4.14 *Jinghua Weikang Jiaowan*

It can regulate Qi to dissipate cold and clear heat and disperse blood stasis. It is usually used for patients with epigastric distension pain or duodenal ulcer caused by mixed coldness and heat syndrome and Qi stagnation and blood stasis and belching; the further symptoms are acid regurgitation, noise, and bitter mouth.

6.4.15 *Ganhai Weikang capsule*

It can strengthen the spleen and stomach and relieve pain with convergence. It was usually used for patients with chronic gastritis stomach and duodenal ulcer and reflux esophagitis caused by spleen deficiency and qi stagnation.

6.4.16 *Dongfang Weiyao capsule*

It can soothe the liver and harmonize stomach, regulate Qi and promote blood circulation, clear heat, and relieve pain. It is usually used for patients with epigastric pain caused by liver-stomach disharmony and heat stasis blocking collaterals; the symptoms are stomachache, belching, acid swallowing, noise, poor appetite, and irritability.

6.4.17 *Yanshen Jianwei capsule*

It can strengthen the spleen and harmonize the stomach, regulate cold and heat, and relieve fullness and pain. It was usually used for patients with stomachache caused by deficiency in origin and enrichment in symptom and mixed coldness and heat; the symptoms are epigastric fullness, stomachache, poor appetite, belching, noise, fatigue, and weakness.

6.4.18 *Danweikang capsule*

It can soothe the liver and gallbladder and clear dampness and heat. It was usually used for patients with hypochondriac pain and jaundice caused by the damp-heat in the liver and gallbladder. It can also be used for patients with bile reflux gastritis and cholecystitis that have the same symptoms.

6.5 Acupuncture and moxibustion therapy

Acupuncture and moxibustion therapy have an effect on improving the symptoms of chronic gastritis. Acupuncture and moxibustion can effectively relieve the symptoms of gastritis in patients with syndrome of deficiency of the spleen and stomach and improve their quality of life [21–24].

Acupoints in acupuncture treatment include Zusanli (ST36), Zhongwan (RN12), Weishu (BL21), Pishu (BL20), and Neiguan (PC6). Patient with liver-stomach disharmony syndrome plus Ganshu (BL17), Taichong (LR4), Qimen (LR14). Patient with hot stasis syndrome plus Tianshu (ST25), Fenglong (ST40). Patient with weakness of spleen and stomach syndrome should add Pishu (BL20), Liang qiu (ST34), Qihai (RN6). Patient with deficiency of stomach Yin syndrome should add Sanyinjiao (SP6), Taixi (KI3). For those with severe cold and deficiency of spleen and stomach syndrome, moxibustion should be performed at Shangwan (RN13), Zhongwan (RN12), Xiawan (RN10), and Zusanli (ST36). Patient with nausea, vomiting, or belching should add Shangwan (RN13), Neiguan (PC6), Geshu (BL17). Patient with severe pain plus Liangmen (ST21), Neiguan (PC6), Gongsun (SP4). Patient with dyspepsia should add Hegu (LI4), Tian shu (ST25), Guanyuan (ST34), Sanyinjiao (SP6). Patient with Qi stagnation and blood stasis syndrome should add Taichong (LR4), Xuehai (SP10), Hegu (LI4). Patient with qi deficiency and blood stasis syndrome should add Xuehai (SP10) and Geshu (BL17). Acupuncture was used for patient with excess syndrome and moxibustion for those with deficiency syndrome. Patient with intermingled deficiency and excess syndrome, acupuncture should combine moxibustion.

6.6 Psychological intervention

Mental stimulation is an important factor causing chronic gastritis, and the scores of anxiety and depression of patients with chronic gastritis are also higher than normal people. Common psychological disorders include loss of confidence in treatment, fear of cancer, and fear of special examinations. Strengthening psychological counseling for gastritis patients is helpful for alleviating the incidence of chronic gastritis, alleviating symptoms, and improving the quality of life [25–27].

7. Criterion of therapeutic effect

7.1 The criteria of therapeutic effect of chronic gastritis include evaluation of syndrome efficacy, symptom evaluation, endoscopic evaluation of gastric mucosa, histopathological evaluation, and evaluation of quality of life

7.1.1 Evaluation of syndrome efficacy

It reflects the characteristics of clinical efficacy evaluation of TCM, and the efficacy is often evaluated by nimodipine method according to the clinical symptoms and manifestations of the tongue and pulse. Clinical recovery: The main symptoms and signs disappear or almost disappear, and the curative effect index was equal or greater than 95%. Significant efficacy: The main symptoms and signs were significantly improved, and curative effect index was equal or greater than 70% or smaller than 95%. Clinical effective: The main symptoms and signs improved, and curative effect index was equal or greater than 30% or smaller than 70%. Ineffectiveness: The main symptoms and signs have no obvious improvement or even worse, curative effect index or smaller than 70%.

7.1.2 Symptom evaluation

It is mainly aimed at the evaluation of dyspepsia symptoms of chronic gastritis, such as upper abdominal pain, fullness or early fullness, loss of appetite, etc. The method was that the symptoms were classified into main symptoms and minor symptoms according to degree and frequency and assign the value according to the weight function, further specification was needed.

7.1.3 Endoscopic evaluation of gastric mucosa

Level I: Branch of Digestive endoscopy of Chinese Medical Association [28] Scattered or discontinuous linear erythema, single erosion, local mucosal hemorrhage, granular gastric mucosal atrophy, partial visible blood vessel, or single gray nodules of intestinal metaplasia. Level II: Dense or continuous linear erythema, more than five local multiple erosion, multiple mucosal hemorrhage, medium gastric mucosal atrophy, continuous visible blood vessel, or multiple gray nodules of intestinal metaplasia. Level III: Extensive fused erythema, more than five extensive multiple erosion, diffuse mucosal hemorrhage, big gastric mucosal atrophy, disappeared mucosal folds, visible blood vessel to mucosa surface, or diffused gray nodules of intestinal metaplasia.

7.1.4 Histopathological evaluation

It includes mucosal trophy, intestinal metaplasia, intraepithelial neoplasia, inflammatory response, and disease activity. They were divided to none, mild level, medium level, and severe level [10]. None level: There are no more than five mononuclear cells in each high-power field. Mild level: There are a few neutrophils in the lamina propria of the gastric mucosa. Chronic inflammatory cells are few and limited to the superficial mucosa, no more than one third of the mucosa. The number of proper mucosal glands decreased by no more than one third of the original glands. Intestinal metaplasia accounts for less than one third of the total glandular and surface epithelial area. Medium level: Neutrophils are more common in the mucosa and can be found in surface epithelial cells, small concave epithelial cells, or glandular epithelium. Chronic inflammatory cells are relatively dense, no more than two thirds of the mucosal layer. The number of proper mucosal glands decreased between one third and two thirds of the original glands. Intestinal metaplasia accounts for one third-two thirds of the total glandular and surface epithelial area. Severe level: The neutrophils are more dense, or pit abscesses may be seen in addition to the medium. Chronic inflammatory cells are dense and occupy the entire mucosal layer. The number of proper glands decreased by more than two thirds, and only a few glands remained or even disappeared completely. Intestinal metaplasia accounts for more than two thirds of the total glandular and epithelial surface area. The visual analogue scoring method combined with histopathological evaluation can be referred to for grading of each lesion.

7.1.5 Evaluation of quality of life

The patient reported outcomes (PRO), and SF-36 health questionnaire scales can be used to evaluate the quality of life. PRO proceeds from the characteristics of TCM treatment of spleen and stomach diseases. Patients were evaluated from six dimensions including dyspepsia, reflux, defecation, social, psychological, and general state [29, 30].

7.1.6 Anxiety and depression evaluation

Hospital anxiety and depression scale (HAD), anxiety self-rating scale (SAS), and depression self-rating scale (SDS) can be used to evaluate the state of anxiety and depression.

7.2 Long-term efficacy

Clinical efficacy evaluation of chronic gastritis should combine short-term efficacy with long-term efficacy evaluation. The course of chronic gastritis is a long-term, chronic, and repeated process. In addition to symptoms, atrophy, intestinal metaplasia, intraepithelial neoplasia, and other lesions should be the important content of observation. The clinical efficacy evaluation time of chronic gastritis is recommended to be more than 3 months in order to accurately evaluate the efficacy. Long-term follow-up was conducted after the treatment to observe the incidence of gastric cancer and other endpoint outcome indicators and disease recurrence.

7.3 Marking targeting biopsy

Marking targeting biopsy of gastric mucosa is of high value for the evaluation of chronic atrophic gastritis and chronic atrophic gastritis with intestinal metaplasia and intraepithelial neoplasia.

8. Prevention and maintenance

8.1 Alimentary control

Research on the relationship between eating behavior and chronic gastritis shows that habits of irregular meals, eating too fast, overeating, eating hot food, eating and drinking too much, salty taste are risk factors for chronic gastritis [29, 30]. Chronic gastritis patients should try to avoid taking stimulating food, such as spicy food, food containing nitrite, etc., and drugs, such as nonsteroidal anti-inflammatory drugs, that may damage the gastric mucosa.

8.2 Psychological adjustment

Patients with chronic gastritis should keep a good mood and avoid the stimulation of bad emotions. If necessary, they can consult a psychologist.

8.3 Lifestyle adjustment

Patients with chronic gastritis should avoid long-term overwork. In winter and spring, we need to pay special attention to life adjustment.

8.4 Follow-up monitoring

Patients with chronic atrophic gastritis accompanied by intraepithelial neoplasia and intestinal metaplasia were followed up and monitored to have a certain probability of cancer. Studies have shown that the time required for 95% of the population with precancerous lesions to become cancerous is 11.6 years for atrophic gastritis, 11.4 years for intestinal metaplasia, 5.7 years for dysplasia, and 4.5 years for moderate to severe intestinal metaplasia with moderate to severe dysplasia [31].

So, the advice of "Chronic gastritis consensus in China" is patients of chronic atrophic gastritis with moderate to severe atrophy and intestinal metaplasia need around 1-year follow-up. Patients of chronic atrophic gastritis without intestinal metaplasia or intraepithelial neoplasia need appropriate follow-up of endoscopy and pathology. Patient accompanied by low-level intraepithelial neoplasia and proved that it doesn't come from adjacent tissues of cancer need once endoscopy every 3 months follow-up according to the endoscopic and clinical situation. However, high-grade intraepithelial neoplasia requires immediate confirmation and endoscopic or surgical treatment after confirmation.

9. Conclusions

The core contents of traditional Chinese medicine (TCM) theory are holism concept and syndrome differentiation; the treatment based on syndrome differentiation is the basic principle of TCM in understanding and treating diseases. So based on the treatment of *Helicobacter pylori* infection, chronic gastritis was treated by Chinese medicine based on disease differentiation. Patients with different syndromes are treated differently with different medicines. Usually, Chinese medicine to treat chronic gastritis is administered orally in decoction or proprietary Chinese medicine. In the recent years, improvement of gastritis drug dosage forms appeared [32], and it was a modern directed drug release preparation with gastric organ flotation and adhesion functions, but more clinical evidence of its effectiveness is lacking.

In conclusion, TCM plays a certain role in improving the clinical symptoms and signs of chronic gastritis. Although the mechanism of its action is not very clear, it still has important clinical value and needs further research and discussion.

Acknowledgements

Authors thank Spleen and Stomach Disease Branch of China Association of Chinese Medicine for the Consensus opinions of TCM diagnosis and treatment experts on chronic gastritis.

Authors thank for the support of National Basic Research Programme of China (973 programme, grant number 2015CB554501).

Conflict of interest

There is no conflict of interest among authors.

Author details

Xiaomei Wang*, Guang Ji and Huangan Wu
Shanghai University of Traditional Chinese Medicine, Shanghai, China

*Address all correspondence to: wxm123@vip.sina.com

References

[1] González CA, Figueiredo C, Lic CB, et al. *Helicobacter pylori* cagA and vacA genotypes as predictors of progression of gastric preneoplastic lesions: A long-term follow-up in a high-risk area in Spain. The American Journal of Gastroenterology. 2011;**106**(5):867-874. DOI: 10.1038/ajg.2011.1

[2] Sharma PK, Suri TM, Venigalla PM, et al. Atrophic gastritis with high prevalence of *Helicobacter pylori* is a predominant feature in patients with dyspepsia in a high altitude area. Tropical Gastroenterology. 2014;**35**(4):246-251

[3] de Vries AC, van Grieken NC, Looman CW, et al. Gastric cancer risk in patients with premalignant gastric lesions: A nationwide cohort study in the Netherlands. Gastroenterology. 2008;**134**(4):945-952. DOI: 10.1053/j.gastro.2008.01.071

[4] Song H, Ekheden IG, Zheng Z, et al. Incidence of gastric cancer among patients with gastric precancerous lesions: Observational cohort study in a low risk Western population. BMJ. 2015;**351**:h3867. DOI: 10.1136/bmj.h3867

[5] Jacobson DL, Gange SJ, Rose NR, Graham NM. Epidemiology and estimated population burden of selected autoimmune diseases in the United States. Clinical Immunology and Immunopathology. 1997;**84**(3):223-243

[6] Song H, Held M, Sandin S, et al. Increase in the prevalence of atrophic gastritis among adults age 35 to 44 years old in Northern Sweden between 1990 and 2009. Clinical Gastroenterology and Hepatology. 2015;**13**(9):1592-1600.e1. DOI: 10.1016/j.cgh.2015.04.001

[7] Spleen and Stomach Disease Branch of China Association of Chinese Medicine. Consensus opinions of TCM diagnosis and treatment experts on chronic gastritis (2017). Chinese Journal of Traditional Chinese Medicine. 2017;**32**(7):3060-3064

[8] Tang XD, Li BS, Zhou LY, et al. Clinical practice guideline of Chinese medicine for chronic gastritis. Chinese Journal of Integrative Medicine. 2012;**18**(1):56-71

[9] Spleen-stomach disease branch of Chinese medical association. Consensus opinions on TCM diagnosis and treatment of chronic atrophic gastritis. Chinese Journal of Integrative Chinese and West Medicine Digestion. 2010;**18**(5):345-349

[10] Gastroenterology breach of Chinese medical association. Consensus on chronic gastritis in China. Chinese Journal of Gastroenterology. 2013;**18**(1):24-36

[11] Xudong T. Academic thoughts on health of Dong Jianhua. Journal of Peking University of Traditional Chinese Medicine. 1995;**18**(2):45-48. DOI: 10.3321/j.issn:1006-2157.1995.02.015

[12] Shengsheng Z. Clinical Study on TCM Syndrome of Chronic Gastritis. Beijing: Peking University of Traditional Chinese Medicine; 2005

[13] Xuewen Z. TCM syndrome treatment of chronic atrophic gastritis. Chinese Archives of Traditional Chinese Medicine. 2002;**20**(5):558-559,587. DOI: 10.3969/j.issn.1673-7717.2002.05.005

[14] Xudong T. Discussion on pathogenesis of blood stasis and treatment of chronic atrophic gastritis. Journal of Traditional Chinese Medicine. 1998;**39**(11):687-689

[15] Li H. Discussion on etiology and pathogenesis of bile reflux gastritis. Shandong Journal of

Traditional Chinese Medicine. 2007;**26**(5):294-295. DOI: 10.3969/j.issn.0257-358X.2007.05.002

[16] Yuyan F, Qian Y, Jianping L, et al. Correlation of syndrome differentiation of TCM and *Helicobacter pylori* infection. Liaoning Journal of Traditional Chinese Medicine. 2005;**32**(8):754-755. DOI: 10.3969/j.issn.1000-1719.2005.08.005

[17] Changhong W, Yuping L, Lixin W, et al. Control observation of correlation between *Helicobacter pylori* infection and inflammatory cell coating on the tongue and syndrome of TCM of 1052 cases of gastritis. Chinese Archives of Traditional Chinese Medicine. 2004;**22**(8):1396-1397. DOI: 10.3969/j.issn.1673-7717.2004.08.017

[18] Suofang S, Weimin L. Professor Shan Zhaowei's experience in treating precancerous lesions of chronic atrophic gastritis. Education of Chinese Medicine. 1998;**17**(4):44-46

[19] Ling H, Jianying M. Professor Lao shaoxian's experience in the diagnosis and treatment of precancerous diseases of gastric cancer. Journal of New Chinese Medicine. 2006;**38**(5):7-9. DOI: 10.3969/j.issn.0256-7415.2006.05.004

[20] Branch of Digestive System Disease of Chinese Association of Integrative Medicine. Consensus on the diagnosis and treatment of chronic gastritis with integrated Chinese and western medicine. Chinese Journal of Integrative Medicine. 2012;**32**(6):738-743

[21] Wenjie J, Lianying C, Jing L, et al. Meta analysis of acupuncture treatment for chronic atrophic gastritis. Shanghai Journal of Acupuncture and Moxibustion. 2016;**35**(7):886-892

[22] Juan X, Zhihui X, Guo C, et al. Meta analysis of acupuncture in the treatment of chronic atrophic gastritis. Guiding Journal of Traditional Chinese Medicine and Pharmacology. 2016;**22**(15):75-78,83

[23] Yinhu X, Xiaoling C. Treating 52 cases of chronic superficial gastritis with deficiency of spleen and stomach. Shaanxi Journal of Traditional Chinese Medicine. 2005;**26**(9):959-960. DOI: 10.3969/j.issn.1000-7369.2005.09.073

[24] Yun Q. Clinical observation on 78 cases of epigastric pain due to deficiency of spleen and stomach with warm acupuncture and ginger moxibustion. Journal of Guiyang College of Traditional Chinese Medicine. 2004;**26**(4):37-38. DOI: 10.3969/j.issn.1002-1108.2004.04.028

[25] Xianling P, Jing M, Houzhi M. Effects of psychological intervention on the curative effect of chronic atrophic gastritis in the elderly. West China Medical Journal. 2014;**29**(4):751-753. DOI: 10.7507/1002-0179.20140226

[26] Xiaoju Z, Xia Z. Effect of nursing intervention on curative effect and mental state of patients with chronic atrophic gastritis. Modern Journal of Integrated Traditional Chinese and Western Medicine. 2015;**24**(10):1130-1132. DOI: 10.3969/j.issn.1008-8849.2015.10.042

[27] Xu J. Effect of comprehensive nursing care on curative effect and mental state of patients with chronic atrophic gastritis. Modern Digestion & Intervention. 2016;**21**(3):492-494. DOI: 10.3969/j.issn.1672-2159.2016.03.047

[28] Branch of Digestive Endoscopy of Chinese Medical Association. Standard of endoscopic classification and classification of chronic gastritis and opinions on trial treatment. Chinese Journal of Digestive Endoscopy. 2004;**21**(2):77-78. DOI: 10.3760/cma.j.issn.1007-5232.2004.02.001

[29] Wei G, Zengzhen W, Xu H, et al. Eating behavior and chronic gastritis. Medicine and Society. 1996;**9**(4):18-19,26

[30] Lan L, Kuicheng Z, Wen W, et al. Case control study on risk factors of chronic atrophic gastritis. Strait Journal Prevetion Medicine. 2016;**22**(4):1-3,7

[31] Shaobo Y, Mengwei W, Ziqi Z, et al. Study on the natural evolution of mucosal changes before gastric cancer. Clinical Medicine of China. 2005;**21**(3):193-194

[32] Lihua L. Research of the Compound Sustained-Release Floating Tablet. Yanji: Yanbian University; 2006

Section 3

Autoimmune Gastritis

Chapter 6

Current View on Autoimmune Gastritis

Mila Dimitrova Kovacheva-Slavova, Todor Asenov Angelov, Hristo Yankov Valkov, Hristo Ilianov Iliev and Borislav Georgiev Vladimirov

Abstract

Autoimmune gastritis (AIG) is a chronic inflammatory disease of the gastric corpus and fundus. Although still unclear, genetic and environmental factors, antigenic mimicry or cross-reactivity are proposed pathogenic mechanisms. Parietal cells destruction results in loss of intrinsic factor and increased gastric pH due to hypochlorhydria and G-cell proliferation. Furthermore, atrophy, intestinal, pancreatic and spasmolytic polypeptide-expressing metaplasia are observed. AIG is underdiagnosed, however, proper diagnostic approach, including endoscopic, serological and histopathological assessment, is required. Gastroscopy with corpus and fundus biopsies is a gold standard. A serological combination of anti-parietal cell antibodies, intrinsic factor antibody, anti-Helicobacter pylori IgG, gastrin, pepsinogen I and pepsinogen I/II ratio improves the diagnostic sensitivity and specificity and allows atrophy level prediction. AIG might manifest with multifactorial iron deficiency anemia, vitamin B12 deficiency (pernicious anemia), neurological and neuropsychiatric conditions, small intestinal bacterial overgrowth and gastrointestinal infections. AIG association with other autoimmune diseases is well-established. Gastric cancer and gastric carcinoid are neoplastic transformations of a continuous chronic inflammation. Patients with AIG should be carefully monitored as no specific AIG therapy is available and disease complication could be fatal.

Keywords: autoimmune gastritis, parietal cells, atrophy, metaplasia, pernicious anemia

1. Introduction

First reported by Thomas Addison (1849) as an atrophic gastritis with autoimmune etiology and co-existing distinctive type of anemia, the autoimmune gastritis (AIG) represents a chronic gastric inflammation with progression to mucosal atrophy, occurring in up to 8% of the general population. Since parietal cells antibodies (PCA) and anti-intrinsic factor antibodies (AIFA) have been first reported by Schwartz (1960) and Irvine (1962), the autoimmune conception of this type of gastritis is recognized. The autoimmune reaction with CD4+ T cells leads to destruction of parietal cells, which are unique cells in the corpus and fundus glands. Therefore, AIG is located in stomach corpus and fundus, which distinguish AIG from other diseases, leading to gastric atrophy (*H. pylori* infection, drugs etc.).

IntechOpen

Based on Sydney System, pyloric or intestinal glands replace the oxyntic glands. The consequences of the loss of parietal cells are hypochlorhydria, gastric pH increasement and decreased production of intrinsic factor with concomitant megaloblastic pernicious anemia in the end-stage due to vitamin B12 malabsorption. Patients might suffer from iron deficiency anemia due to hypochlorhydria and inadequate iron uptake. Gastrointestinal symptoms are rarely reported. AIG is often presented with other autoimmune co-morbidities (thyroid autoimmune disease, type 1 diabetes, etc.). Although gastrointestinal symptoms are rarely reported, a malignant transformations, namely intestinal-type gastric cancer and type I gastric carcinoid are observed in respectively 5.3% and ca. 9% of AIG patients [1–3].

2. Epidemiology

Nowadays the prevalence of AIG is difficult to obtain, as the disease occurs asymptomatic in early stages, remains undiagnosed for a long period as symptoms arise with atrophy and mucosal dysplasia progression. Further explanations for the underdiagnosed AIG are the inadequate and not from the right location biopsy sampling and the poor identification of the etiology of anemia, which is one of the AIG manifestations. Estimated incidence is ca. 2% in younger and up to 12% in elderly patients. Studies demonstrate increased prevalence of AIG with advancing age and in patients with *H. pylori* infection (Zhang et al.). Females are more often affected than males (3:1 ratio), although this has not been consistently observed. Cabreta et al. in their randomized study find no age difference. The reported prevalence of pernicious anemia, which is one of the most typical AIG manifestations, is about 0.1% in the general population and about 2% in elderly (older than 60 years). The prevalence of pernicious anemia does not differ between populations (white, African American and non-white Hispanic). A study of Carmel and Johnson elucidate that African American women develop pernicious anemia at significantly younger age. Association with other autoimmune diseases (autoimmune thyroid diseases - Hashimoto's thyroiditis and Graves' disease, type 1 diabetes, vitiligo, Addison's disease etc.) is documented to additionally increase the prevalence to up to 35%. This consequence determines a multiple autoimmune diseases (MAS) type 3B and 4. Pernicious anemia is present in patients with Graves' disease, Hashimoto's thyroiditis, type 1 diabetes, autoimmune thyroid disease, Addison's disease, primary hypoparathyroidism and vitiligo in 2, 4–12%, up to 4, 2–12, 6, 9 and 3–8%, respectively. Recent data direct the attention to the possible association between *H. pylori* infection and AIG development in respect to molecular mimicry between *H. pylori* antigens and the gastric H+/K+ adenosine-triphosphate enzyme (ATPase). Few studies evaluate the incidence of AIG (using histology, PCA positive levels) in patients with iron deficiency anemia (IDA) of unknown etiology. The estimated prevalence varies between 15 and 27%. The profile of patients with IDA and positive PCA are younger females with lower hemoglobin and ferritin levels and who suffer more often from restless legs syndrome [1, 2, 4–14].

3. Pathogenesis

AIG is a chronic inflammation, localized in the gastric corpus and fundus. The inflammatory processes start with lymphocytes and plasma cells infiltration in lamina propria with involvement of deep layers, leading to parietal cells destruction. Because of preservation of relatively normal oxyntic mucosa, a gastric pseudopolyposis appears (also known as "islands in the sea"). The loss of parietal cells results in hypochlorhydria and further in G-cell hyperplasia due to missing negative feedback, leading to higher gastrin secretion in the antrum. A further consequence of the increased gastric pH is the parietal cell pseudohypertrophy. The higher gastrin secretion leads to direct stimulation of enterochromaffin-like (ECL) cells and their proliferation in hyperplastic, dysplastic and neoplastic subtypes that might onset a carcinoid tumor. Pseudopyloric metaplasia ("oxyntic antralization", spasmolytic polypeptide-expressing metaplasia (SPEM)), intestinal metaplasia (IM) and pancreatic metaplasia can be observed. SPEM can be transformed into IM, which represents the replacement of gastric mucosa with intestinal epithelium (small intestinal and colonic). AIG results in microcytic iron deficiency anemia and megalocytic pernicious anemia due to vitamin B12 deficiency [2, 4].

3.1 Immunogenetic factors

AIG and PCA are observed in 20–30% of the family members of patients with pernicious anemia. However, a genetic predisposition has been proposed. Although the association between pernicious anemia and particular HLA haplo/genotypes is weak, studies evaluate HLA DR4, with DR2 and DR5 haplotypes. A genetic heterogeneity is observed in respect to DR3/DR4 genotype, which is found in patients with pernicious anemia and concomitant endocrinopathy. Using murine models, 4 distinct genetic regions of susceptibility genes for AIG were identified (Gasa1, 2, 3 and 4) on chromosomes 4 and 6 and H2 region. Interestingly, three of these genes are nonmajor histocompatibility complex genes and are located on the same locus with those of type 1 diabetes, which could explain the strong concordance between AIG and type 1 diabetes [2, 15–18].

3.2 Cell-mediated autoimmunity

Cell-mediated autoimmunity has a key role for the AIG development. The main trigger of autoimmunity are the 100-kd catalytic α-subunit and the 60- to 90-kd glycoprotein β-subunit of the gastric H+/K + -ATPase, which membrane protein is a proton pump. PCA and AIFA are found in both serum and gastric juice. The higher the PCA titer is, the more severe the corpus atrophy is and the lower the parietal cells concentration is. The loss of parietal cells is a consequence of mainly CD4+ CD25− Th1 resting lymphocyte effectors initiated perforin-mediated cytotoxicity (perforin/granzyme B pathway) or Fas–FasL apoptosis. CD4+ CD25− Th1 resting lymphocyte effectors produce IFN-γ and TNF-α. Submucosa, lamina propria and gastric glands are infiltrated by CD4 + CD25− T-cells, together with macrophages and B lymphocytes, leading to loss of parietal (CD4+ T cells react to H+/K+-ATPase α chain and marginally to the β chain), principal and P/D1 ghrelin-producing cells [2, 5, 15, 19–21].

3.3 Humoral autoimmunity

Two types of antibodies are produced by B cells from activated CD4+ T cells in patients with AIG, namely PCA (antibody to the parietal cells) and AIFA (antibody to the produced by the parietal cells a 60-kDa glycoprotein intrinsic factor). PCA are found in the serum and gastric juice in up to 90% and AIFA in 30–50% of AIG patients. A catalytic and β subunits of gastric H+/K + -ATPase are bound by PCA. In end-stages of AIG the PCA titer decreases because of parietal cells loss. Researchers have found two types of AIFA from IgG class. Type 1 is present in 70% of patients and acts as a blocking antibody that reacts with the binding site for vitamin B12. Type 2 AIFA is present in 30% of patients and is a precipitating antibody that binds other binding sites from vitamin B12 and impedes binding of intrinsic factor-vitamin B12 to the receptors in the ileal mucosa [5, 22–24].

3.4 Association with *H. pylori*

H. pylori, which is well-established etiological factor for atrophic gastritis development, may induce AIG through mechanisms of molecular mimicry at the T-cell level (autoreactive T cells against gastric proton pump), bystander activation and / or epitope spreading. This hypothesis is supported by recent studies as some patients may have AIG with co-existing *H. pylori* infection (20–50%). *H. pylori* leads to development of various antibodies, including PCA and anticanalicular antibodies against the H+/K+ ATPase, which are in fact most frequent. Studies show a high homology between the β subunit of *H. pylori* urease and the subunit β of gastric proton pump, which is a precondition for cross-reactivity against parietal cells and IFN-γ production, resulting in killing or apoptotic suicide. Some patients with PCA and/or AIFA, who underwent *H. pylori* eradication, demonstrated loss of antigastric antibodies. However, the correlation between AIG and *H. pylori* still remains controversial. AIG patients with observed gastric atrophy or IM in the course of *H. pylori* infection do not decrease their risk for gastric cancer development even after *H. pylori* eradication [2, 5, 25–30].

3.5 Endocrine factors

AIG is frequently associated with other autoimmune diseases. Emphasized is the link to type 1 diabetes and autoimmune thyroid disease (Hashimoto's thyroiditis and Graves' disease). Reported risk factors for patients with AIG and type 1 diabetes are persistent positive islet cell antibody and positive glutamic acid decarboxylase-65 antibody, which is found in the thyroid gland and stomach except in pancreas and brain. Studies demonstrate that type 1 diabetes itself and not hereditary might be a risk factor for AIG development. Positive thyroid peroxidase autoantibody are reported in up to 50%of AIG patients due to possible cross-reaction. As PCA are verified in up to 40% of patients with autoimmune thyroid diseases, screening the patients of this population for AIG should be recommended. Other reported co-existing autoimmune conditions are polyglandular autoimmune syndromes (mainly type 3B), Addison's disease, vitiligo, perioral cutaneous autoimmune diseases (mainly erosive oral lichen) and myasthenia gravis [2, 4, 7, 31–34].

4. Diagnostic approach

4.1 Serological tests

The evaluation of AIG-associated autoantibodies (PCA and AIFA), anti-*H. pylori* antibodies (anti-HP-IgG) and markers for gastric atrophy (gastrin and pepsinogen levels) is used for serological noninvasive diagnosis of AIG ("serological biopsy", the so-called GastroPanel test (ELISA test, Biohit, Helsinki, Finland)). AIG-associated autoantibodies are widely used for screening and diagnosis of AIG. They differ according to their sensitivity and specificity as PCA is higher sensitive (80% compared to 50% sensitivity for AIFA) but less specific for pernicious anemia detection. Studies are controversial whether PCA levels correlate with AIG severity or not. Due to low gastric acid output and G-cells stimulation and elevated gastrin secretion in patients with atrophic autoimmune gastritis, it is crucial to evaluate gastrin levels (usually gastrin 17) as gastrin correlates strong with gastric atrophy based on histopathology. Other useful atrophy markers are the produced by the chief cells of oxyntic mucosa of stomach corpus and fundus pepsinogen I and the secreted by the chief cells and mucous neck cells of the whole stomach mucosa pepsinogen II. In patients with atrophic autoimmune gastritis are demonstrated significant decrease of pepsinogen I (low pepsinogen II levels are not commonly observed) and low Pepsinogen I/Pepsinogen II ratio (<3). In respect to diagnosis of pernicious anemia, a panel of vitamin B12, homocysteine and methylmalonic acid measurement is required. In those patients may be observed thrombocytopenia, increased levels of LDH and bilirubin, and rarely schistocytes in the peripheral smear. Iron deficiency anemia, which is often present in patients with AIG, should be identified by levels of hemoglobin, mean corpuscular volume (MCV), serum iron, ferritin, total iron-binding capacity (TIBS) and serum transferrin receptor (TfR). In patients with suspected carcinoid tumor transformation the measurement of chromogranin A, which is secreted by the ECL cells, can be useful, although it shows low specificity (23%) and false-positive results in patients with inflammatory bowel disease, renal insufficiency and other conditions [4, 23, 35–45].

4.2 Endoscopy

Of a great importance for AIG diagnosis is the performance of gastroscopy with separately collected biopsies - two from the corpus, two from the antrum and one from the incisura angularis (updated Sydney System recommendations). New endoscopic techniques (magnifying endoscopy, autofluorescence and narrow-band imaging) improve the diagnostic accuracy as they provide information for minimal gastric atrophic changes. A number of endoscopic appearances can be present: polyps (hyperplastic or adenomatous), pseudopolyps, flattened rugal folds, visible submucosal vessels, loss of subepithelial capillary network resembling honeycomb, collecting venules in regular shape and appearance and vascular pattern and swelling of areae gastricae. A combination of them improves the sensitivity and specificity of the procedure. In early AIG stages with minimal or no endoscopical and histological changes, gastric acid production is increased due to hypo- or achlorhydria. Thus, gastric acid measurement (simple intragastric pH measurement or volume of acid secretion) might be useful for early AIG diagnosis [1, 4, 46–52].

4.3 Histopathology

Histopathological assessment of biopsies form gastric corpus and fundus remains gold standard for AIG diagnosis even in early stages of the disease. The correct site of biopsy is of great importance for the proper AIG diagnosis, which could be tested by immunohistochemical staining of G cells (gastrin). Histological characteristics change with disease progression. Typical but non-specific for AIG are lymphoplasmacytic infiltration in lamina propria, which is mainly multifocal with accentuation in the deeper; glandular portion in early stage and diffuse lymphoplasmacytic infiltration of the lamina propria in end-stage; focal to profound atrophy of oxyntic mucosa with disease progression. End-stage AIG is further characterized by distinct reduction or total loss of oxyntic glands with pseudohypertrophy of parietal cells due to fragmentary oxyntic glands destruction in end-stage of AIG; SPEM presence; pancreatic or intestinal metaplasia; ECL cells hyperplasia with additional samples immunohistochemical testing with chromogranin A and synaptophysin [1, 4, 11, 53–57].

5. Clinical presentation

Symptoms vary during the course of AIG as patients at early stages are most often asymptomatic, which makes the diagnostic approach only on clinical presentation challenging. With disease progression a wide spectrum of gastrointestinal, hematological and neurological signs and symptoms arises [1, 3, 4].

5.1 Gastrointestinal manifestations

Gastrointestinal symptoms are not the leading presentation of patients with AIG. Carabotti et al. report in their recent study frequency of one or more gastrointestinal symptoms in 56.7% of AIG patients. Female gender, younger age (<55 years) and non-smoking are independent risk factors for gastrointestinal symptoms manifestation. More than half of the patients had upper gastrointestinal complains as most frequent one was vague dyspepsia in respect to post-prandial fullness and/or early satiation. Furthermore, as achlorhydria is a major pathogenetic consequence of AIG, patients may suffer from bloating, delayed gastric emptying, small intestinal bacterial overgrowth, and gastrointestinal infections such as *Clostridium difficile*. Pain and peptic or duodenic ulcers are not reported. Atrophic glossitis due to vitamin B12 deficiency is an early stage AIG manifestation. Interestingly, heartburn (24%) and acid regurgitation (12%) are presented in a study of Miceli et al., which could develop from nonacidic refluxes. Data exist to support the observation that gastroesophageal reflux disease and its complications like Barrett's esophagus may develop even in AIG patients [1–4, 6, 58–69].

5.2 Hematological manifestations

Typical hematological manifestations of AIG are iron deficiency anemia (IDA) in the early stages and pernicious anemia in the end-stage of the disease.

IDA is the leading hematological manifestation, occurring in 50% of AIG patients as reported by Hershko et al. Several epidemiological studies demonstrate IDA in younger patients prior to pernicious anemia development. Iron metabolism, which is regulated by an uptake, is impaired in AIG mainly due to the presence of achlorhydria. Different mechanisms of IDA with AIG etiology are observed. For the necessary reduction of the ferric form of inorganic iron (the iron type in food) to ferrous as well as for releasing the ferric/ferrous iron from its protein-complex in order to precede to an iron uptake, gastric acid is needed. Another cause for IDA in AIG is the decreased iron absorption due to lack of ascorbic acid, destroyed in AIG. IDA symptoms vary as the commonly reported are fatigue, brittle nails, hair loss, restless legs syndrome, immune dysfunction, ineffective wound healing, while due to anemia itself tachycardia, shortness of breath, dizziness, lightheadedness and cognitive and physical dysfunction may develop. Pregnant women are at risk of early birth and underweight newborns. Of great importance is that IDA with AIG etiology is refractory to iron therapy [1, 4, 6, 13, 20, 58–60, 70–75].

Pernicious anemia is usually caused by vitamin B12 deficiency due to loss of intrinsic factor and insufficient releasing of vitamin B12 from the food due to low levels of gastric acid. Vitamin B12 is a key regulator of DNA synthesis. Mostly affected are patients at advanced age due to age-related reduced absorption and minimal turnover with further large stores of vitamin B12. The clinical manifestations vary widely; therefore pernicious anemia is so-called "great pretender". Reported symptoms of pernicious anemia are fatigue, lightheadedness, palpitations, angina pectoris and congestive heart failure and mental disturbances. Patients are at increased risk of endovascular dysfunction and myocardial infarction and pulmonary embolism due to hyperhomocysteinemia and the related thrombosis. Therefore, untreated pernicious anemia may lead to lethal exit [1, 4, 6, 20, 58–61, 76–80].

5.3 Neurological manifestations

Neuronal death due to demyelination and axonal damage leads to the typical neurological manifestation of vitamin B12, which might be present even in patients with no hematological changes. The loss of vibratory and position sensations together with distal paresthesias develop from damages in the lateral and posterior columns of the cervical and upper thoracic segments of the spinal cord. This syndrome is called a subacute combined degeneration and is very specific for pernicious anemia. Other vitamin B12 deficiency presentations are peripheral neuropathy (paresthesia and numbness of the lower extremities), optic neuropathy and neuropsychiatric conditions (dementia, mania, depression, psychosis, obsessive–compulsive disorder, etc.). Proper diagnosis and early vitamin B12 substitution are mandatory to delay progression and for better outcome [1, 4, 81–89].

6. Neoplastic transformations

Patients with AIG are at increased risk of gastric cancer development. The estimated prevalence is about 5.3% as recent studies suggest even higher incidence - 14.2 per 1000 person-years with patients with AIG having risk of gastric cancer development 3 to 6-fold higher than the general population. Recent meta-analysis demonstrates 0.27% per person-year with an overall relative risk of 6.8 (95% CI 2.6–18.1) for gastric cancer development. Elderly people, chronic inflammation due to *H. pylori* infection, achlorhydria, presence of dysplasia and intestinal metaplasia are significantly risk factors for gastric tumorogenesis [1, 57, 90].

6.1 Gastric carcinoid

Gastric carcinoids are verified in 4–9% of patients with AIG and pernicious anemia. 50–85% of all gastric carcinoids develop in patients with AIG. Three types of gastric carcinoids are established, of which type I is found in patients with AIG, type II is associated with Zollinger-Ellison syndrome and multiple endocrine neoplasia I and type III carcinoid is the most aggressive type. Achlorhydria is a key factor for the development of gastric carcinoids in AIG patients. As described, achlorhydria leads to loss of negative feedback and G-cells stimulation in antrum, followed by hypergastrinemia (typical for type I and II carcinoids). The high gastrin levels demonstrate trophic effects on ECL cells hyperplasia, which further may result in dysplasia and transformation into gastric carcinoid. Gastric carcinoids are quite benign lesions with low metastatic potential (less than 10%). Patients with gastric carcinoids are usually asymptomatic. However, they may complain of dyspepsia, abdominal pain, flushing, diarrhea and symptoms of anemia. Classical carcinoid syndrome is seen very rare. Carcinoids are usually diagnosed incidentally during endoscopy in patients with anemia. Gastroscopy with biopsy sampling with further immunostaining for chromogranin A and/or neuron-specific enolase is the best diagnostic approach. The presence of polyps in the stomach body in patients with AIG is significantly associated with type I carcinoid. As long as polyps might be underdiagnosed during endoscopy, serum chromogranin A levels are more accurate for carcinoids diagnosis. Chromogranin A levels correlate strong with gastrin levels and ECL cell density in the corpus and fundus mucosa, representing high specificity (59%) and sensitivity (100%). According to the algorithm of Gilligan et al. based on size and number, gastric carcinoids in AIG patients, which size is <1 cm and the number is 3–5, should be removed endoscopically, and those >1 cm and/or > 5 should be followed by antrectomy. Surveillance at every 6-month is proposed. Another therapeutic option is the administration of octreotide, which leads to lower gastrin levels, improved ECL status and even spontaneous regression (Ferraro et al.) [1, 2, 4, 45, 90–110].

6.2 Gastric cancer

The chronic inflammation, which is an integral part of the pathogenesis of AIG, increases significantly the risk of malignant transformations. Achlorhydria, high dietary salt intake and bacterial overgrowth are proposed risk factors. Furthermore, the concomitant *H. pylori* infection additionally increases the risk of precancerous lesions. Current studies suggest that cancer stem cells, which might be exposed on mutations, have an important role in cancerogenesis. This concept is assumed as stem cells are well-known for their longevity and inherent capacity for self-renewal. As a consequence of chronic inflammation, stem cells level and proliferation potential increase, which favors their intestinal metaplasia (possible phenotype of stem cells abnormality) and dysplasia. In 1988, Correa and Piazuelo proposed the so-called "Correa hypothesis/cascade" for gastric cancer development in patients with *H. pylori* infection: unknown genetic and epigenetic factors lead stepwise to 1. chronic inflammation; 2. atrophy gastritis; 3. intestinal metaplasia; 4. low to high grade dysplasia, which finally results in gastric cancer in some patients. *H. pylori* factors, associated with higher malignancy potential are CagA-positive strains, VacA gene and s1 m1 [1, 4, 5, 111–120].

An attention is paid at the role of tumor-associated autoantigens in immunogenicity and immunodiagnosis, which may detect cancer at early stage. Usually these autoantigens are cellular proteins, which can be ectopically expressed or a result from genetic mutations and rearrangements. Additional mutations in the tumor-associated autoantigens lead to new antigenic epitopes and finally increased immunogenicity. According to a current concept of the immunological response of cancer tissue, tumor-associated antigens lead to autoantibodies production. Autoantibodies with potential clinical usefulness are anti-carcinoembryonic antigen (CEA), anti-p53, anti-survivin, anti-mucin, and anti-livin autoantibodies. The autoantibodies are missing in healthy people and non-cancer diseases. Thus, autoantibodies against tumor antigens can serve as biomarkers and may have the potential to verify an early stage cancer, which may significantly improve patients diagnosis and outcome as the majority of patients with gastric cancer are diagnosed late, when are symptomatic and the management is rather palliative. Studies show significant lower levels of biomarkers after radical tumor resection, which suggest their prominent role in patient monitoring [5, 121–125].

The estimated frequency of detection of anti-carcinoembryonic antigen (CEA) anti-survivin, anti-mucin, and anti-livin autoantibodies is 46–56, 40, 75 and 50%, respectively, as anti-CEA is found in 10% of healthy people. They are present in the early stage of gastric cancer and demonstrate a good prognostic value for survival and postoperative monitoring, especially in patients without anti-p53 antibodies [123, 126–131].

p53 is a key factor in carcinogenesis. In 46% of patients with p53-positive gastric cancer are found increased anti-p53 antibodies levels. Anti-p53 antibodies, which are first reported in patients with breast cancer, correlate significantly with the tumor suppressor gene p53 protein expression, demonstrating about 96% specificity for neoplastic detection. In contrast to anti-carcinoembryonic antigen (CEA) anti-survivin, anti-mucin, and anti-livin autoantibodies, anti-p53 antibodies are not appropriate markers for early diagnosis and prognosis as they are detected in advanced gastric tumors with regional lymph node involvement [123, 126, 132–134].

Extracellular protein kinase A (ECPKA) is a cAMP-dependent intracellular enzyme. Anti- ECPKA antibodies are significantly increased in patients with gastric cancer and other malignancies. They have the potential to be future universal screening method for tumors of different origin as their sensitivity and specificity are very high - 90 and 87%, respectively [135].

The presence of substantial number heterogeneous autoantibodies varies widely and demonstrates high specificity but low diagnostic sensitivity. To improve their sensitivity in order to enable their application in clinical practice for screening and diagnosis of gastric cancer; it is reasonable to promote a combination of serological AIG- and tumor biomarkers, microRNAs and/or glycosylation signatures. Using a combination of 5 biomarkers (MAGEA4, CTAG1, TP53, ERBB2_C, and SDCCAG8), Werner et al. demonstrated 32% sensitivity and 87% specificity for diagnosis of early stage gastric adenocarcinoma. In a study of Zhou et al. a combination of 7 markers, namely p53, Koc, p62, c-myc, IMP1, survivin and p16, identified gastric cancer with sensitivity and specificity of 64% and 87%, respectively. Wang et al. verified a panel of 8 biomarkers (IMP1, p62, Koc, p53, c-myc, cyclin B1, survivin and p16), able to detect gastric cancer with 56.1% sensitivity and 86.2% specificity [136–144].

7. Treatment

Up-to-date there is no consensus on whom to screen for AIG and how often. The treatment management of AIG with avoiding further complications requires according to the present symptoms, serological results and imaging data proper follow-up. A proper monitoring with testing once a year complete blood count, gastrin, iron and vitamin B12 levels seems to be beneficial. Therapy depends on the stage of AIG, *H. pylori* infection, current nutrient deficiencies, concomitant autoimmune conditions and (pre)malignant transformation. As described above, *H. pylori* infection may play a crucial role in AIG pathogenesis. However, screening for *H. pylori* (serological anti-HP-Ig G and Ig M, fecal HP-antigen, breath tests, histological and cultural methods) in patients with AIG, gastric atrophy, intestinal metaplasia/dysplasia, and hypo- or achlorhydria should be performed. If positive for *H. pylori*, patients need subsequent treatment and eradication. Studies support *H. pylori* treatment as *H. pylori* eradication was associated with decreased levels of PCA and AIFA and AIG early stages healing. Oral supplementation with vitamin B12, iron and folic acid is recommended in early stages of AIG. With neurological symptoms occurring, parenteral vitamin B12 should be applied. As long as various autoimmune diseases are recognized as AIG co-morbidities, attention should be paid at their screening and following treatment. Researchers recommend the routine screening for type 1 diabetes and autoimmune thyroid diseases. On the other hand, in patients, who are diagnosed with type 1 diabetic (positive glutamate decarboxylase-65 antibodies) and autoimmune thyroiditis (positive thyroid peroxidase antibodies), PCA should be investigated at the disease's onset and thereafter yearly for 3 years and later on a longer intervals if there is no AIG clinical signs. Screening for AIG in those patients' populations might avoid the development of IDA and pernicious anemia with their above mentioned serious complications. As long as gastric carcinoid is curative, proper diagnosis and radical treatment are essential. According to size, number and location of gastric cancer / carcinoid, polypectomy, antrectomy (gastrin-producing part), surgical eradication of a gastric tumor, with resection of adjacent lymph nodes or medicamentous treatment with further surveillance is performed. Somatostatin analogs are used as they can reduce gastrin and chromogranin A levels in patients with neuroendocrine tumor (carcinoid). Promising therapeutic option is the gastrin receptor antagonist Netazepide, leading to decreased chromogranin A levels together with cancer size and number. A new technique for carcinoid tumors treatment is the peptide receptor radiotherapy, which would be worth to be tested in AIG patients. Whether to perform surveillance program with regular endoscopic and histological examination in patients with AIG or not remains controversial and guidelines according to AIG surveillance are missing. If mild to moderate dysplasia or ECL cell hyperplasia are observed, an endoscopic surveillance every 5 years is proposed. In contrast to the rare and with far better prognosis carcinoids, gastric cancer development might be fatal. According to the American Society for Gastrointestinal Endoscopy recommendations (2006) for monitoring of patients with *H. pylori* atrophic gastritis, depending on the primary endoscopic finding the follow-up should be in intervals of 3–5 years (patients with simple, linear/micronodular hyperplasia); every 3 years (patients with extensive atrophy/IM) or every year (patients with adenomas/low-grade dysplasia) [1, 2, 11, 90, 103, 109, 113, 145–153].

8. Discussion

Although *H. pylori* is a leading cause for gastritis, AIG frequency is increasing in elderly people and in those with other autoimmune pathology. As AIG is commonly underdiagnosed, AIG should be considered in the differential diagnosis of patients with anemia, dyspepsia and especially in those with concomitant autoimmune thyroid disease and type 1 diabetes and with relatives with gastric neoplasia. *H. pylori* presence does not exclude AIG in the pathogenesis of an underlying gastritis. Screening of patients with a panel of serological markers pepsinogen I and II, gastrin, and/or *H. pylori* antibodies as well as the antibodies PCA and AIFA directs to the need of gastroscopy. However, gastroscopy with separately collected biopsies and histopathological assessment of specimens form gastric corpus and fundus remain the gold standard for AIG diagnosis. Asymptomatic in the early stages of the disease, AIG is not recognized in guidelines as an etiological factor for iron deficiency. However, AIG is often leading to iron deficiency anemia, which requires a different treatment strategy. Untreated pernicious anemia, which is a later manifestation of AIG, could cause both neurological complications and letal cardiovascular events. AIG is a precancerosis for the development of gastric cancer and neuroendocrine tumors. An effort is required to identify a biomarker panel with high sensitivity for early-stage gastric malignancy diagnosis. The treatment of AIG still remains challenging due to asymptomatic early stage and complex pathogenesis of the disease.

9. Conclusion

Proper and early diagnostic approach and prevention, followed by patients' carefully lifelong monitoring at yearly intervals is mandatory to improve the prognosis and outcome of AIG. New therapeutic strategies are needed to delay disease progression and influence the gastric atrophy, making it a reversible entity. Guidelines of AIG surveillance are awaited.

Acknowledgements

The publication of this work was supported by Vladimir Jeglov and Valeri Andreev.

DOI: http://dx.doi.org/10.5772/intechopen.87006

Conflict of interest

There is no conflict.

Author details

Mila Dimitrova Kovacheva-Slavova[1*], Todor Asenov Angelov[1], Hristo Yankov Valkov[1], Hristo Ilianov Iliev[2] and Borislav Georgiev Vladimirov[1]

1 Department of Gastroenterology, University Hospital "Tsaritsa Ioanna-ISUL", Medical University of Sofia, Sofia, Bulgaria

2 Medical University of Sofia, Sofia, Bulgaria

*Address all correspondence to: kovacheva_mila@abv.bg

References

[1] Kulnigg-Dabsch S. Autoimmune gastritis. Autoimmungastritis. Wiener Medizinische Wochenschrift. 2016;**166**(13-14):424-430. DOI: 10.1007/s10354-016-0515-5

[2] De Block CEM, De Leeuw IH, Van Gaal LF. Autoimmune gastritis in type 1 diabetes: A clinically oriented review. The Journal of Clinical Endocrinology & Metabolism. 2008;**93**(2):363-371. DOI: 10.1210/jc.2007-2134

[3] Carabotti M, Lahner E, Esposito G, Sacchi MC, Severi C, Annibale B. Upper gastrointestinal symptoms in autoimmune gastritis: A cross-sectional study. Medicine. 2017;**96**(1):e5784. DOI: 10.1097/MD.0000000000005784

[4] Minalyan A, Benhammou JN, Artashesyan A, Lewis MS, Pisegna JR. Autoimmune atrophic gastritis: Current perspectives. Clinical and Experimental Gastroenterology. 2017;**10**:19-27. DOI: 10.2147/CEG.S109123

[5] Bizzaro N, Antico A, Villalta D. Autoimmunity and gastric cancer. International Journal of Molecular Sciences. 2018;**19**(2):377. DOI: 10.3390/ijms19020377

[6] Hershko C et al. Variable hematologic presentation of autoimmune gastritis: Age-related progression from iron deficiency to cobalamin depletion. Blood. 2006;**107**(4):1673-1679

[7] Zhang Y et al. Gastric parietal cell antibodies, helicobacter pylori infection, and chronic atrophic gastritis: Evidence from a large population-based study in Germany. Cancer Epidemiology, Biomarkers & Prevention. 2013;**22**(5):821-826

[8] Kulnigg-Dabsch S et al. Autoimmune gastritis is common in patients with iron deficiency – Non-invasive evaluation of iron deficiency aside guideline recommendations. Gastroenterology. 2015;**148**(4):1

[9] Carmel R, Johnson CS. Racial patterns in pernicious anemia. Early age at onset and increased frequency of intrinsic-factor antibody in black women. The New England Journal of Medicine. 1978;**298**(12):647-650

[10] Lam-Tse WK, Batstra MR, Koeleman BP, et al. The association between autoimmune thyroiditis, autoimmune gastritis and type 1 diabetes. Pediatric Endocrinology Reviews. 2003;**1**(1):22-37

[11] Neumann WL, Coss E, Rugge M, Genta RM. Autoimmune atrophic gastritis – Pathogenesis, pathology and management. Nature Reviews Gastroenterology & Hepatology. 2013;**10**(9):529-541

[12] Dickey W et al. Gastric as well as duodenal biopsies may be useful in the investigation of iron deficiency anaemia. Scandinavian Journal of Gastroenterology. 1997;**32**(5):469-472

[13] Annibale B et al. Gastrointestinal causes of refractory iron deficiency anemia in patients without gastrointestinal symptoms. The American Journal of Medicine. 2001;**111**(6):439-445

[14] Kaye PV et al. The clinical utility and diagnostic yield of routine gastric biopsies in the investigation of iron deficiency anemia: A case-control study. The American Journal of Gastroenterology. 2008;**103**(11):2883-2889

[15] De Block CE, De Leeuw IH, Van Gaal LF. High prevalence of manifestations of gastric autoimmunity in parietal cell antibody-positive type 1 (insulin-dependent) diabetic patients. The Belgian diabetes registry. The

Journal of Clinical Endocrinology and Metabolism. 1999;**84**:4062-4067

[16] Baxter AG, Jordan MA, Silveira PA, Wilson WE, van Driel IR. Genetic control of susceptibility to autoimmune gastritis. International Reviews of Immunology. 2005;**24**:55-62

[17] van Driel IR, Baxter AG, Laurie KL, Zwar TD, La Gruta NL, Judd LM, et al. Immunopathogenesis, loss of T cell tolerance and genetics of autoimmune gastritis. Autoimmunity Reviews. 2002;**1**:290-297

[18] van Driel IR, Read S, Zwar T, Gleeson PA. Shaping the T cell repertoire to a bona fide autoantigen: Lessons from autoimmune gastritis. Current Opinion in Immunology. 2005;**17**:570-576

[19] D'Elios MM, Bergman MP, Azzurri A, Amedei A, Benagiano M, de Pont JJ, et al. H(+),K(+)- ATPase (proton pump) is the target autoantigen of Th1-type cytotoxic T cells in autoimmune gastritis. Gastroenterology. 2001;**120**:377-386. DOI: 10.1053/gast.2001.21187

[20] Toh BH, Van Driel IR, Gleeson PA. Mechanisms of disease: Pernicious anemia. The New England Journal of Medicine. 1997;**337**:1441-1448. DOI: 10.1056/NEJM199711133372007

[21] Callaghan JM, Khan MA, Alderuccio F, van Driel IR, Gleeson PA, Toh BH. Alpha and beta subunits of the gastric H+/K+-ATPase are concordantly targeted by parietal cell autoantibodies associated with autoimmune gastritis. Autoimmunity. 1993;**16**:289-295. DOI: 10.3109/08916939309014648

[22] Toh BH, Alderuccio F. Pernicious anaemia. Autoimmunity. 2004;**37**: 357-361. DOI: 10.1080/0891693 0410001705439

[23] Antico A, Tampoia M, Villalta D, Tonutti E, Tozzoli R, Bizzaro N. Clinical usefulness of the serological gastric biopsy for the diagnosis of chronic autoimmune gastritis. Clinical & Developmental Immunology. 2012;**2012**:520970. DOI: 10.1155/ 2012/520970

[24] Tozzoli R, Kodermaz G, Perosa AR, Tampoia M, Zucano A, Antico A, et al. Autoantibodies to parietal cells as predictors of atrophic body gastritis: A five-year prospective study in patients with autoimmune thyroid diseases. Autoimmunity Reviews. 2010;**10**:80-83. DOI: 10.1016/j.autrev.2010.08.006

[25] Weck MN, Brenner H. Association of helicobacter pylori infection with chronic atrophic gastritis: Meta-analyses according to type of disease definition. International Journal of Cancer. 2008;**123**:874-881. DOI: 10.1002/ijc.23539

[26] Claeys D, Faller G, Appelmelk B, Negrini R, Kirchner T. The gastric H+/ K+ ATPase is a major autoantigen in chronic helicobacter pylori gastritis with body mucosa atrophy. Gastroenterology. 1998;**115**:340-347. DOI: 10.1016/ S0016-5085(98)70200-8

[27] Amedei A, Bergman MP, Appelmelk B, Azzurri A, Benagiano M, Tamburini C, et al. Molecular mimicry between helicobacter pylori antigens and H+K+-adenotriphosphatase in human gastric autoimmunity. The Journal of Experimental Medicine. 2003;**198**:1147-1156. DOI: 10.1084/jem.20030530

[28] D'Elios MM, Appelmelk BJ, Amedei A, Bergman MP, Del Prete GF. Gastric autoimmunity: The role of helicobacter pylori and molecular mimicry. Trends in Molecular Medicine. 2004;**10**:316-323. DOI: 10.1016/j.molmed.2004.06.001

[29] Veijola LI, Oksanen AM, Sipponen PI, Rautelin HIK. Association of autoimmune type atrophic corpus gastritis with helicobacter pylori infection. World Journal of Gastroenterology. 2010;**16**(1):83-88

[30] Faller G, Steininger H, Eck M, Hensen J, Hann EG, Kirchner T. Anti-gastric autoantibodies in helicobacter pylori gastritis: Prevalence, in-situ binding sites and clues for clinical relevance. Virchows Archiv. 1996;**427**(5):483-486

[31] Massironi S, Zilli A, Elvevi A, Invernizzi P. The changing face of chronic autoimmune atrophic gastritis: an updated comprehensive perspective. Autoimmunity Reviews. 2019;**18**(3):215-222. DOI: 10.1016/j.autrev.2018.08.011

[32] Venerito M, Radünz M, Reschke K, Reinhold D, Frauenschläger K, Jechorek D, et al. Autoimmune gastritis in autoimmune thyroid disease. Alimentary Pharmacology & Therapeutics. 2015;**41**:686-693. DOI: 10.1111/apt.13097

[33] Checchi S, Montanaro A, Ciuoli C, et al. Prevalence of parietal cell antibodies in a large cohort of patients with autoimmune thyroiditis. Thyroid. 2010;**20**:1385-1389

[34] Castoro C, Le Moli R, Arpi ML, et al. Association of autoimmune thyroid diseases, chronic atrophic gastritis and gastric carcinoid: Experience from a single institution. Journal of Endocrinological Investigation. 2016;**39**(7):779-784

[35] Rusak E, Chobot A, Krzywicka A, Wenzlau J. Anti-parietal cell antibodies – diagnostic significance. Advances in Medical Sciences. 2016;**61**(2):175-179

[36] Khan S, Del-Duca C, Fenton E, et al. Limited value of testing for intrinsic factor antibodies with negative gastric parietal cell antibodies in pernicious anaemia. Journal of Clinical Pathology. 2009;**62**(5):439-441

[37] Phan J, Benhammou JN, Pisegna JR. Gastric hypersecretory states: Investigation and management. Current Treatment Options in Gastroenterology. 2015;**13**(4):386-397

[38] Carmel R. Pepsinogens and other serum markers in pernicious anemia. American Journal of Clinical Pathology. 1988;**90**(4):442-445

[39] Noah D, Assoumou M, Bagnaka S, Ngaba G, Alonge I, Paloheimo L, et al. Assessing GastroPanel serum markers as a non-invasive method for the diagnosis of atrophic gastritis and helicobacter pylori infection. Open Journal of Gastroenterology. 2012;**2**:113-118. DOI: 10.4236/ojgas.2012.23024

[40] Storskrubb T, Aro P, Ronkainen J. Serum biomarkers provide an accurate method for diagnosis of atrophic gastritis in a general population: The Kalixanda study. Scandinavian Journal of Gastroenterology. 2008;**43**:448-1455

[41] Syrjänen K. Serological biomarker panel (GastroPanel®): A test for non-invasive diagnosis of dyspeptic symptoms and for comprehensive detection of helicobacter pylori infection. Biomark J. 2017;**3**:1

[42] Väänänen H, Vauhkonen M, Helske T. Non-endoscopic diagnosis of atrophic gastritis with a blood test. Correlation between gastric histology and serum levels of gastrin-17 and pepsinogen I: A multicenter study. European Journal of Gastroenterology & Hepatology. 2003;**15**:885-891

[43] Syrjänen K. A panel of serum biomarkers (GastroPanel®) in non-invasive diagnosis of atrophic gastritis. Systematic review and meta-analysis. Anticancer Research. 2016;**36**:5133-5144

[44] Solomon LR. Cobalamin-responsive disorders in the ambulatory care setting: Unreliability of cobalamin, methylmalonic acid, and homocysteine testing. Blood. 2005;**105**(3):978-985

[45] Wu PB, Deng YZ, Shu YX, Tan SY, Li M, Fang G. Increased plasma CgA levels associated with nonalcoholic fatty

liver disease. The Turkish Journal of Gastroenterology. 2015;**26**(5):404-407

[46] Nomura S, Ida K, Terao S, et al. Endoscopic diagnosis of gastric mucosal atrophy: Multicenter prospective study. Digestive Endoscopy. 2014;**26**(6):709-719

[47] Park YH, Kim N. Review of atrophic gastritis and intestinal metaplasia as a premalignant lesion of gastric cancer. Journal of Cancer Prevention. 2015;**20**(1):25-40

[48] Anagnostopoulos GK, Ragunath K, Shonde A, Hawkey CJ, Yao K. Diagnosis of autoimmune gastritis by high resolution magnification endoscopy. World Journal of Gastroenterology. 2006;**12**(28):4586-4587

[49] Dai Y-C, Tang Z-P, Zhang Y-L. How to assess the severity of atrophic gastritis. World Journal of Gastroenterology. 2011;**17**(13):1690-1693

[50] Toh BH. Diagnosis and classification of autoimmune gastritis. Autoimmunity Reviews. 2014;**13**(4-5):459-462

[51] Okano A, Takakuwa H, Matsubayashi Y. Parietal-cell hyperplasia mimicking sporadic fundic gland polyps in the atrophic mucosa of autoimmune gastritis. Gastrointestinal Endoscopy. 2007;**66**(2):394-395

[52] Ghosh T et al. Review article: Methods of measuring gastric acid secretion. Alimentary Pharmacology & Therapeutics. 2011;**33**(7):768-781

[53] Park JY, Lam-Himlin D, Vemulapalli R. Review of autoimmune metaplastic atrophic gastritis. Gastrointestinal Endoscopy. 2013;**77**(2):284-292

[54] Pittman ME et al. Autoimmune metaplastic atrophic gastritis: Recognizing precursor lesions for appropriate patient evaluation. The American Journal of Surgical Pathology. 2015;**39**(12):1611-1620

[55] Wong HH, Chu P. Immunohisto-chemical features of the gastrointestinal tract tumors. Journal of Gastrointestinal Oncology. 2012;**3**(3):262-284

[56] Sepulveda AR, Patil M. Practical approach to the pathologic diagnosis of gastritis. Archives of Pathology & Laboratory Medicine. 2008;**132**(10):1586-1593

[57] Joo YE, Park HK, Myung DS, Baik GH, Shin JE, Seo GS, et al. Prevalence and risk factors of atrophic gastritis and intestinal metaplasia: A nationwide multicenter prospective study in Korea. Gut and Liver. 2013;**7**(3):303-310. DOI: 10.5009/gnl.2013.7.3.303

[58] Lahner E, Carabotti M, Annibale B. Atrophic body gastritis: Clinical presentation, diagnosis, and outcome. EMJ Gastroenterology. 2017;**6**(1):75-82

[59] Miceli E, Lenti MV, Padula D, Luinetti O, Vattiato C, Monti CM, et al. Common features of patients with autoimmune atrophic gastritis. Clinical Gastroenterology and Hepatology. 2012;**10**(7):812-814. DOI: 10.1016/j.cgh.2012.02.018

[60] Hershko C, Patz J, Ronson A. The anemia of achylia gastrica revisited. Blood Cells, Molecules & Diseases. 2007;**39**(2):178-183

[61] Lahner E, Annibale B. Pernicious anemia: New insights from a gastroenterological point of view. World Journal of Gastroenterology. 2009;**15**(41):5121-5128

[62] Zhu JC, Wang YF, Sheng J, Chen FX, Tang GY. Atrophic glossitis is attributed to cobalamin deficiency. Shanghai J Stomatol. 2013;**22**(1):58-62

[63] Soykan I, Yakut M, Keskin O, et al. Clinical profiles, endoscopic and laboratory features and associated factors in patients with autoimmune gastritis. Digestion. 2012;**86**:20-26

[64] Tenca A, Massironi S, Pugliese D, et al. Gastro-esophageal reflux and antisecretory drugs use among patients with chronic autoimmune atrophic gastritis: A study with pH-impedance monitoring. Neurogastroenterology and Motility. 2016;**28**:274-280

[65] Vakil N, van Zanten SV, Kahrilas P, et al. Global consensus group the Montreal definition and classification of gastroesophageal reflux disease: A global evidence-based consensus. The American Journal of Gastroenterology. 2006;**101**:1900-1920

[66] Tack J, Talley NJ, Camilleri M, et al. Functional gastroduodenal disorders. Gastroenterology. 2006;**130**:1466-1479

[67] Carabotti M, Lahner E, Severi C, et al. A case of Barrett's oesophagus in pernicious anaemia: Acid is not the only culprit! Therapeutic Advances in Gastroenterology. 2016;**9**:419-421

[68] Kalkan Ç, Soykan I, Soydal Ç, et al. Assessment of gastric emptying in patients with autoimmune gastritis. Digestive Diseases and Sciences. 2016;**61**:1597-1602

[69] Iwai W, Abe Y, Iijima K, et al. Gastric hypochlorhydria is associated with an exacerbation of dyspeptic symptoms in female patients. Journal of Gastroenterology. 2013;**48**:214-221

[70] Bezwoda W et al. The importance of gastric hydrochloric acid in the absorption of nonheme food iron. The Journal of Laboratory and Clinical Medicine. 1978;**92**(1):108-116

[71] Cook JD, Brown GM, Valberg LS. The effect of Achylia Gastrica on iron absorption. The Journal of Clinical Investigation. 1964;**43**:1185-1191

[72] Aditi A, Graham DY. Vitamin C, gastritis, and gastric disease: A historical review and update. Digestive Diseases and Sciences. 2012;**57**(10):2504-2515

[73] Hershko C, Hoffbrand A, Keret D, et al. Role of autoimmune gastritis, helicobacter pylori and celiac disease in refractory or unexplained iron deficiency anemia. Haematologica. 2005;**90**(5):585-595

[74] Gonçalves C, Oliveira ME, Palha AM, Ferrão A, Morais A, Lopes AI. Autoimmune gastritis presenting as iron deficiency anemia in childhood. World Journal of Gastroenterology. 2014;**20**(42):15780-15786

[75] Annibale B, Capurso G, Delle Fave G. The stomach and iron deficiency anaemia: A forgotten link. Digestive and Liver Disease. 2003;**35**:288-295

[76] Stabler SP. Clinical practice. Vitamin B12 deficiency. The New England Journal of Medicine. 2013;**368**(2):149-160

[77] Asimacopoulos PJ, Groves MD, Fischer DK, et al. Pernicious anemia manifesting as angina pectoris. Southern Medical Journal. 1994;**87**(6):671-672

[78] Tadakamalla AK, Talluri SK, Besur S. Pseudo-thrombotic thrombocytopenic purpura: A rare presentation of pernicious anemia. North American Journal of Medical Sciences. 2011;**3**(10):472-474

[79] Shamkani WA, Jafar NS, Narayanan SR, Rajappan AK. Acute myocardial infarction in a young lady due to vitamin B12 deficiency induced hyperhomocysteinemia. Heart Views. 2015;**16**(1):25-29

[80] Whittingham S, Mackay IR. Pernicious anemia and gastric atrophy. In: Rose NR, Mackay IR, editors. The Autoimmune Diseases. New York: Academic Press; 1985. pp. 243-266

[81] Metz J. Cobalamin deficiency and the pathogenesis of nervous system disease. Annual Review of Nutrition. 1992;**12**:59-79

[82] Francis G, Hohol K, Jawad Z, Ayer A, Toth C. Methylmalonic acid accumulation and the development of peripheral neuropathy (IN1-1.010). Neurology. 2012;**78**(1 suppl):IN1-IN1

[83] Ralapanawa DM, Jayawickreme KP, Ekanayake EM, Jayalath WA. B(12) deficiency with neurological manifestations in the absence of anaemia. BMC Research Notes. 2015;**8**:458

[84] Lindenbaum J, Healton EB, Savage DG, et al. Neuropsychiatric disorders caused by cobalamin deficiency in the absence of anemia or macrocytosis. The New England Journal of Medicine. 1988;**318**(26):1720-1728

[85] Vasconcelos OM, Poehm EH, McCarter RJ, Campbell WW, Quezado ZMN. Potential outcome factors in subacute combined degeneration: Review of observational studies. Journal of General Internal Medicine. 2006;**21**(10):1063-1068

[86] Saperstein DS, Barohn RJ. Peripheral neuropathy due to cobalamin deficiency. Current Treatment Options in Neurology. 2002;**4**(3):197-201

[87] Chu C, Scanlon P. Vitamin B12 deficiency optic neuropathy detected by asymptomatic screening. BML Case Reports. 2011;**2011**:bcr0220113823

[88] Metzler D, Miller WH, Stephen EC. Psychiatric manifestation of vitamin B-12 deficiency: An update. Jefferson Journal of Psychiatry. 1991;**9**(2)

[89] Douaud G, Refsum H, de Jager CA, et al. Preventing Alzheimer's disease-related gray matter atrophy by B-vitamin treatment. Proceedings of the National Academy of Sciences of the United States of America. 2013;**110**(23):9523-9528

[90] Mahmud N, Stashek K, Katona BW, Tondon R, Shroff SG, Roses R, et al. The incidence of neoplasia in patients with autoimmune metaplastic atrophic gastritis: A renewed call for surveillance. Annals of Gastroenterology. 2018;**32**(1):67-72. DOI: 10.20524/aog.2018.0325

[91] Kokkola A, Sjöblom SM, Haapiainen R, Sipponen P, Puolakkainen P, Jarvinen H. The risk of gastric carcinoma and carcinoid tumours in patients with pernicious anaemia: A prospective follow-up study. Scandinavian Journal of Gastroenterology. 1998;**33**:88-92

[92] De Block CE, De Leeuw IH, Pelckmans PA, Michielsen PP, Bogers JJ, Van Marck EA, et al. Autoimmune hepatitis, autoimmune gastritis, and gastric carcinoid in a type 1 diabetic patient: A case report. Journal of Diabetes and its Complications. 2000;**14**:116-120

[93] De Block CE, Colpin G, Thielemans K, Coopmans W, Bogers JJ, Pelckmans PA, et al. Neuroendocrine tumor markers and enterochromaffin-like cell hyper/dysplasia in type 1 diabetes. Diabetes Care. 2004;**27**(6):1387-1393

[94] Modlin IM, Kidd M, Latich I, Zikusoka MN, Shapiro MD. Current status of gastrointestinal carcinoids. Gastroenterology. 2005;**128**:1717-1751

[95] Vannella L et al. Development of type I gastric carcinoid in patients with chronic atrophic gastritis. Alimentary Pharmacology & Therapeutics. 2011;**33**(12):1361-1369

[96] Rindi G, Luinetti O, Cornaggia M, Capella C, Solcia E. Three subtypes of gastric argyrophil carcinoid and the gastric neuroendocrine carcinoma: A clinicopathologic study. Gastroenterology. 1993;**104**:994-1006

[97] Gough DB, Thompson GB, Crotty TB, Donohue JH, Kvols LK, Carney A, et al. Diverse clinical and pathologic features of gastric carcinoid and the relevance of hypergastrinemia. World Journal of Surgery. 1994;**18**:473-479

[98] Borch K, Stridsberg M, Burman P, Rehfeld JF. Basal chromogranin A and gastrin concentrations in circulation correlate to endocrine cell proliferation in type A gastritis. Scandinavian Journal of Gastroenterology. 1997;**32**:198-202

[99] Borch K, Renvall H, Liedberg G. Gastric endocrine cell hyperplasia and carcinoid tumors in pernicious anemia. Gastroenterology. 1985;**88**:638-648

[100] Peracchi M, Gebbia C, Basilisco G, Quatrini M, Tarantino C, Vescarelli S, et al. Plasma chromogranin A in patients with autoimmune chronic atrophic gastritis, enterochromaffin-like cell lesions and gastric carcinoids. European Journal of Endocrinology. 2005;**152**:443-448

[101] Sjöblom SM, Sipponen P, Jarvinen H. Gastroscopic follow-up of pernicious anaemia patients. Gut. 1993;**34**:28-32

[102] Hirschowitz BI, Griffith J, Pellegrin D, Cummings OW. Rapid regression of enterochromaffinlike cell gastric carcinoids in pernicious anemia after antrectomy. Gastroenterology. 1992;**102**(4 Pt 1):1409-1418

[103] Ferraro G, Annibale B, Marignani M, Azzoni C, D'Adda T, D'Ambra G, et al. Effectiveness of octreotide in controlling fasting hypergastrinemia and related enterochromaffin-like cell growth. The Journal of Clinical Endocrinology and Metabolism. 1996;**81**:677-683

[104] Zhou K, Ho W. Gastric carcinoids: Classification and diagnosis. In: Pisegna RJ, editor. Management of Pancreatic Neuroendocrine Tumors. New York, NY: Springer New York; 2015. pp. 83-93

[105] Burkitt MD, Pritchard DM. Review article: Pathogenesis and management of gastric carcinoid tumours. Alimentary Pharmacology & Therapeutics. 2006;**24**(9):1305-1320

[106] Li T-T, Qiu F, Qian ZR, Wan J, Qi X-K, Wu B-Y. Classification, clinicopathologic features and treatment of gastric neuroendocrine tumors. World Journal of Gastroenterology. 2014;**20**(1):118-125

[107] Creutzfeldt W. The achlorhydria-carcinoid sequence: Role of gastrin. Digestion. 1988;**39**(2):61-79

[108] Bordi C et al. Hypergastrinemia and gastric enterochromaffin-like cells. The American Journal of Surgical Pathology. 1995;**19**(Suppl 1):S8-S19

[109] Nikou GC, Angelopoulos TP. Current concepts on gastric carcinoid tumors. Gastroenterology Research and Practice. 2012;**2012**:287825

[110] Vanoli A, La Rosa S, Luinetti O, Klersy C, Manca R, Alvisi C, et al. Histologic changes in type A chronic atrophic gastritis indicating increased risk of neuroendocrine tumor development: The predictive role of dysplastic and severely hyperplastic enterochromaffin-like cell lesions. Human Pathology. 2013;**44**:1827-1837. DOI: 10.1016/j.humpath.2013.02.005

[111] Correa P. A human model of gastric carcinogenesis. Cancer Research. 1988;**48**(13):3554-3560

[112] Vannella L et al. Systematic review: Gastric cancer incidence in pernicious anaemia. Alimentary Pharmacology & Therapeutics. 2013;**37**(4):375-382

[113] Hirota WK et al. ASGE guideline: The role of endoscopy in the surveillance of premalignant conditions of the upper GI tract. Gastrointestinal Endoscopy. 2006;**63**(4):570-580

[114] Schneller J, Gupta R, Mustafa J, Villanueva R, Straus EW, Raffaniello RD. Helicobacter pylori infection is associated with a high incidence of intestinal metaplasia in the gastric mucosa of patients at inner-city hospitals in New York. Digestive Diseases and Sciences. 2006;**51**(10):1801-1809

[115] Wong BC, Lam SK, Wong WM, et al. China gastric cancer study group helicobacter pylori eradication to prevent gastric cancer in a high-risk region of China: A randomized controlled trial. Journal of the American Medical Association. 2004;**291**(2):187-194

[116] Correa P, Piazuelo MB. The gastric precancerous cascade. Journal of Digestive Diseases. 2012;**13**(1):2-9

[117] Yong X, Tang B, Li B-S, et al. Helicobacter pylori virulence factor CagA promotes tumorigenesis of gastric cancer via multiple signaling pathways. Cell Communication and Signaling: CCS. 2015;**13**(1):1-13

[118] Van Doorn LJ, Figueiredo C, Sanna R, Plaisier A, Schneeberger P, de Boer W, et al. Clinical relevance of the cagA, vacA, and iceA status of helicobacter pylori. Gastroenterology. 1998;**115**:58-66. DOI: 10.1016/S0016-5085(98)70365-8

[119] Yamaoka Y. Mechanisms of disease: Helicobacter pylorivirulence factors. Nature Reviews Gastroenterology & Hepatology. 2010;**7**(11):629-641

[120] Wroblewski LE, Peek RM, Wilson KT. Helicobacter pylori and gastric cancer: Factors that modulate disease risk. Clinical Microbiology Reviews. 2010;**23**(4):713-739

[121] Tan EM. Autoantibodies as reporters identifying aberrant cellular mechanisms in tumorigenesis. Journal of Clinical Investigation. 2001;**108**:1411-1415. DOI: 10.1172/JCI14451

[122] Werner S, Chen H, Tao S, Brenner H. Systematic review: Serum autoantibodies in the early detection of gastric cancer. International Journal of Cancer. 2015;**136**:2243-2252. DOI: 10.1002/ijc.28807

[123] Macdonald IK, Parsy-Kowalska CB, Chapman CJ. Autoantibodies: Opportunities for early cancer detection. Trends in Cancer. 2017;**3**:198-213. DOI: 10.1016/j.trecan.2017.02.003

[124] Liu W, Peng B, Lu Y, Xu W, Qian W, Zhang JY. Autoantibodies to tumor-associated antigens as biomarkers in cancer immunodiagnosis. Autoimmunity Reviews. 2011;**10**:331-335. DOI: 10.1016/j.autrev.2010.12.002

[125] Zaenker P, Ziman MR. Serologic autoantibodies as diagnostic cancer biomarkers—A review. Cancer Epidemiology, Biomarkers & Prevention. 2013;**22**:2161-2181. DOI: 10.1158/1055-9965.EPI-13-0621

[126] Konstadoulakis MM, Syrigos KN, Albanopoulos C, Mayers G, Golematis B. The presence of anti-carcinoembryonic antigen (CEA) antibodies in the sera of patients with gastrointestinal malignancies. Journal of Clinical Immunology. 1994;**14**:310-313. DOI: 10.1007/BF01540984

[127] Saif MW, Zalonis A, Syrigos K. The clinical significance of autoantibodies in gastrointestinal malignancies: An overview. Expert Opinion on Biological Therapy. 2007;**7**:493-507. DOI: 10.1517/14712598.7.4.493

[128] Ura Y, Ochi Y, Hamazu M, Ishida M, Nakajima K, Watanabe T. Studies on circulating antibody against carcinoembryonic antigen (CEA) and CEA-like antigen in cancer patients. Cancer Letters. 1985;**25**:283-295. DOI: 10.1016/S0304-3835(15)30008-2

[129] Albanopoulos K, Armakolas A, Konstadoulakis MM, Leandros E, Tsiompanou E, Katsaragakis S, et al. Prognostic significance of circulating antibodies against carcinoembryonic antigen (anti-CEA) in patients with colon cancer. The American Journal of Gastroenterology. 2000;**95**:1056-1061. DOI: 10.1111/j.1572-0241.2000.01982.x

[130] Nakamura H, Hinoda Y, Nakagawa N, Makiguchi Y, Itoh F, Endo T, et al. Detection of circulating anti-MUC1 mucin core protein antibodies in patients with colorectal cancer. Journal of Gastroenterology. 1998;**33**:354-361. DOI: 10.1007/s005350050096

[131] Yagihashi A, Asanuma K, Nakamura M, Araya J, Mano Y, Torigoe T, et al. Detection of anti-survivin antibody in gastrointestinal cancer patients. Clinical Chemistry. 2001;**47**:1729-1731

[132] Flammann HT, Kuhn HM. P53 autoantibodies and cancer: Specificity, diagnosis and monitoring. In: Shoenfeld Y, Gershwin ME, editors. Cancer and Autoimmunity. Amsterdam, The Netherlands: Elsevier Science; 2000. pp. 181-188

[133] Soussi T. p53 antibodies in the sera of patients with various types of cancer: A review. Cancer Research. 2000;**60**:1777-1788

[134] Shimada H, Ochiai T, Nomura F. Japan p53 antibody research group. Titration of serum p53 antibodies in 1085 patients with various types of malignant tumors: A multiinstitutional analysis by the Japan p53 antibody research group. Cancer. 2003;**97**:682-689. DOI: 10.1002/cncr.11092

[135] Cho-Chung YS. Autoantibody biomarkers in the detection of cancer. Biochimica et Biophysica Acta. 2006;**1762**:587-591. DOI: 10.1016/j.bbadis.2006.04.001

[136] Qiu LL, Hua PY, Ye LL, Wang YC, Qiu T, Bao HZ, et al. The detection of serum anti-p53 antibodies from patients with gastric carcinoma in China. Cancer Detection and Prevention. 2007;**31**:45-49. DOI: 10.1016/j.cdp.2006.12.005

[137] Zhou SL, Ku JW, Fan ZM, Yue WB, Du F, Zhou YF. Detection of autoantibodies to a panel of tumor-associated antigens for the diagnosis values of gastric cardia adenocarcinoma. Diseases of the Esophagus. 2015;**28**:371-379. DOI: 10.1111/dote.12206

[138] Shimizu K, Ueda Y, Yamagishi H. Titration of serum p53 antibodies in patients with gastric cancer: A single-institute study of 40 patients. Gastric Cancer. 2005;**8**:214-219. DOI: 10.1007/s10120-005-0337-4

[139] Wang P, Song C, Xie W, Ye H, Wang K, Dai L, et al. Evaluation of diagnostic value in using a panel of multiple tumor-associated antigens for immunodiagnosis of cancer. Journal of Immunology Research. 2014;**2014**:512540. DOI: 10.1155/2014/512540

[140] Shimada H, Noie T, Ohashi M, Oba K, Takahashi Y. Clinical significance of serum tumor markers for gastric cancer: A systematic review of literature by the task force of the Japanese gastric cancer association. Gastric Cancer. 2014;**17**:26-33. DOI: 10.1007/s10120-013-0259-5

[141] Werner S, Chen H, Butt J, Michel A, Knebel P, Holleczek B, et al. Evaluation of the diagnostic value of 64 simultaneously measured

autoantibodies for early detection of gastric cancer. Scientific Reports. 2016;**6**:25467. DOI: 10.1038/srep25467

[142] Di Mario F, Cavallaro LG. Non-invasive tests in gastric diseases. Digestive and Liver Disease. 2008;**40**:523-530. DOI: 10.1016/j.dld.2008.02.028

[143] Majeed W, Iftikhar A, Khaliq T, Aslam B, Muzaffar H, Atta K, et al. Gastric carcinoma: Recent trends in diagnostic biomarkers and molecular targeted therapies. Asian Pacific Journal of Cancer Prevention. 2016;**17**:3053-3060

[144] Zayakin P, Ancāns G, Siliņa K, Meistere I, Kalniņa Z, Andrejeva D, et al. Tumor-associated autoantibody signature for the early detection of gastric cancer. International Journal of Cancer. 2013;**132**:137-147. DOI: 10.1002/ijc.27667

[145] Dinis-Ribeiro M et al. Management of precancerous conditions and lesions in the stomach (MAPS): Guideline from the European Society of Gastrointestinal Endoscopy (ESGE), European Helicobacter Study Group (EHSG), European Society of Pathology (ESP), and the Sociedade Portuguesa de Endoscopia Digestiva (SPED). Endoscopy. 2012;**44**(1):74-94

[146] Andres E, Fothergill H, Mecili M. Efficacy of oral cobalamin (vitamin B12) therapy. Expert Opinion on Pharmacotherapy. 2010;**11**(2):249-256

[147] Stolte M, Meier E, Meining A. Cure of autoimmune gastritis by helicobacter pylori eradication in a 21-year-old male. Zeitschrift für Gastroenterologie. 1998;**36**(8):641-643

[148] Faller G, Winter M, Steininger H, et al. Decrease of antigastric autoantibodies in helicobacter pylori gastritis after cure of infection. Pathology, Research and Practice. 1999;**195**(4):243-246

[149] Dockray GJ. Clinical endocrinology and metabolism. Gastrin. Best Practice & Research Clinical Endocrinology & Metabolism. 2004;**18**(4):555-568

[150] Moore AR, Boyce M, Steele IA, Campbell F, Varro A, Pritchard DM. Netazepide, a gastrin receptor antagonist, normalises tumour biomarkers and causes regression of type 1 gastric neuroendocrine tumours in a nonrandomised trial of patients with chronic atrophic gastritis. PLoS One. 2013;**8**(10):e76462

[151] Kwekkeboom DJ, Krenning EP. Peptide receptor radionuclide therapy in the treatment of neuroendocrine tumors. Hematology/Oncology Clinics of North America. 2016;**30**(1):179-191

[152] Fossmark R, Sordal O, Jianu CS, et al. Treatment of gastric carcinoids type 1 with the gastrin receptor antagonist netazepide (YF476) results in regression of tumours and normalisation of serum chromogranin A. Alimentary Pharmacology & Therapeutics. 2012;**36**(11-12):1067-1075

[153] Massironi S, Zilli A, Fanetti I, Ciafardini C, Conte D, Peracchi M. Intermittent treatment of recurrent type-1 gastric carcinoids with somatostatin analogues in patients with chronic autoimmune atrophic gastritis. Digestive and Liver Disease. 2015;**47**(11):978-983